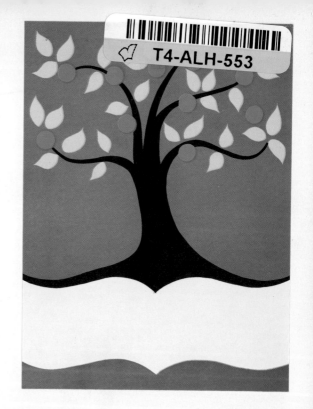

Veterinary
Medical Mycology

PAUL F. JUNGERMAN, D.V.M., M.S.

Formerly Professor, Veterinary Microbiology, Texas A & M University;
Pet Medical Clinic, Austin, Texas

ROBERT M. SCHWARTZMAN, V.M.D., Ph.D.

School of Veterinary Medicine, University of Pennsylvania, Philadelphia,
Pennsylvania

Veterinary Medical Mycology

Lea & Febiger

Philadelphia · 1972

To Evelyn Lee

ISBN 0–8121–0322–X

Library of Congress Catalog Card Number: 78–157469

Printed in the United States of America

Preface

This book is an outgrowth of our lectures to students of veterinary medicine and medical mycology given over the past fifteen years. During this time, we have recognized the need for a textbook devoted exclusively to the animal mycoses. Knowledge of the pathogenic fungi and the diseases they cause has accumulated very rapidly during the past two decades. Prior to that time mycology was a neglected and little understood science in most teaching programs, often without recognition or departmental affiliation. As the mycoses were discovered with increasing frequency and their importance more fully realized, mycology has attained a status as a medical specialty. As curriculum changes have come about, this specialty has gradually received more time both in basic science and clinical teaching.

In the past few years some useful and some promising therapeutic agents have been discovered. It is hopefully anticipated that others, especially for treatment of the deep mycoses, will emerge from the search for more effective antibiotics. More precise criteria for the identification of the fungi have been discovered. New culture media have been developed and, in combination with improved methods of culture, have given the mycologist a new efficiency. Whenever applicable, we have attempted to merge this information with our own clinical and laboratory observations.

We have prepared the format with the veterinary medical student in mind. It was designed for use in the classroom and laboratory; we hope it will have supplemental use in pathology and clinical medicine. Also, we endeavored to make it useful to diversified interests in the veterinary profession: practitioners, epidemiologists, and researchers.

Believing it is more properly taught in toxicology courses, we have omitted a discussion of mycotoxicosis. Also omitted are rare and doubtful mycotic diseases. Some are so rare that adequate descriptions are impossible; others lack authenticity. In time, some will no doubt be found important; but until more cases and reports can be reviewed, we prefer omission to inadequacy.

Although knowledge of medical mycology has accumulated very rapidly, there are still gaps and voids. Certain areas are controversial. In these we have usually taken a stand, because we think it is better for students to fix to a speculative fact than to half accept two conflicting opinions. Hopefully we will not be considered overly didactic, for we know that eventually new information will show us to be wrong in some cases.

Debts of gratitude are owed to many friends and colleagues for encouragement and help in preparation of the manuscript. Included are many of the teaching and research faculty of our respective veterinary colleges, Texas A & M University and The University of Pennsylvania. Drs. G. M. Gowing, C. H. Bridges, and T. J. Galvin contributed unusual aid and counsel. A special tribute is due the late Dr. Hilton A. Smith who was colleague, friend, and teacher to one of us (P.F.J.). In one or two cases, his descriptions of pathologic changes were so clear and instructional that they were quoted verbatim.

Austin, Texas   PAUL F. JUNGERMAN
Philadelphia, Pa.   ROBERT M. SCHWARTZMAN

Contents

Part I
THE DERMATOPHYTOSES

CHAPTER 1

Microsporosis and Trichophytosis

Dermatomycosis (Ringworm)

Dermatomycosis (ringworm) is an integumentary disease caused by fungi belonging to a group referred to as dermatophytes.* These organisms, when living on the host, inhabit and are limited to the most superficial parts of the body, viz., the keratin of the stratum corneum, nails, and hair. They are non-invasive, cannot survive in living tissue, nor in areas of intense inflammation, and they have keratolytic activity.[1] Ringworm has been reported in all species of domesticated animals.

HISTORY, GEOGRAPHIC DISTRIBUTION AND PREVALENCE

Of the mycotic diseases affecting animals and man, ringworm was the first to be recognized and reported. The medical history of the disease is not only the oldest, but also the most voluminous and contains such eminent names as Gruby and Sabouraud. In 1843, Gruby named *Microsporum audouinii* as a causative agent of ringworm in children; two years later, Lebert described the causative agent of favus, *Trichophyton schoenleinii* (cited by Emmons and co-workers).[2] Infection in chickens by *Trichophyton gallinae* was reported in 1881,[3] *Trichophyton mentagrophytes* infection in cattle in 1894,[4] *Microsporum canis* infection in horses and dogs in 1896 and 1897[5,6] and *Trichophyton equinum* infection in horses in 1898.[7] Sabouraud's monumental work which classified and brought order to the dermatophytic group was published in 1910.[8] Since that time, thousands of reports of ringworm infections in animals have appeared in the veterinary and medical literature. Extensive reviews of this literature have been written by Blank,[9] Georg[10] and Dawson.[11]

Ringworm has a worldwide geographic distribution. The disease appears to be more common in tropical and temperate climates, and particularly in countries or

---

* The probable place of origin of all dermatophytes is the soil. A significant number of organisms have given up their saprophytic existence in nature for a parasitic existence on animal or human skin. On the basis of the preferential habitat of the dermatophytes, the organisms may be classified as geophilic (soil loving) or keratinophilic (keratin loving). Further classification of the dermatophytes has been made on the basis of (1) preference of the organism for human or animal tissue (anthropophilic or zoophilic); (2) position of the fungal spores on or in the hair (ectothrix or endothrix); (3) cultural characteristics; and (4) in man, the position on the body which is preferentially affected (tinea capitis, tinea barbae, tinea corporis).

TABLE 1–1. Tentative Diagnosis of Ringworm in Animals from Clinical Materials*

Fungus Species	Animals Affected	Location and Appearance of Lesions	Wood's Light Examination	Direct Examination in KOH Mounts	
				Skin Scrapings	Hair
		MICROSPORUM INFECTIONS			
Microsporum canis	COMMON: Cats Dogs OCCASIONAL: Horses Monkeys RARE: Rabbits Rodents Chinchillas	Scattered lesions, but especially on head. Adult cats and dogs: infections may be clinically inapparent, or may be represented by loss of hair only. Young animals: lesions usually more clearly defined. Discrete circular areas of hair loss with scaling and occasionally inflamed borders are common. Heavy crusts may develop in these areas. Severe clinical cases may appear in both young and adult animals, with heavy crusted areas or widespread loss of hair, scaling and erythema. Horse: lesions particularly in harness areas ("girth itch")	Bright yellow green fluorescence of infected hairs	Mycelium and chains of arthrospores	Sheath of small spores (2–3μ) in mosaic, completely surrounds hair at base. Easily dislodged from hair in preparation. Mycelium within hair running parallel to its length.
Microsporum gypseum	COMMON: Dogs OCCASIONAL: Cats Horses Wild rodents	Infection may be clinically inapparent. Often a single lesion on head or leg or scattered discrete lesions over body. Circular areas with loss of hair and some scaliness, or heavy yellowish brown crusts which later fall off leaving a "moth-eaten" appearance to animal. Hairs loose at edges of crusts. Some hairs embedded in crusts	No fluorescence	Mycelium and masses of very large arthrospores, some in chains	Large spores (5–8μ) in chains or in irregular masses on surface of hairs. Mycelium within hair, running parallel to its length

Microsporum audouinii	RARE: Dogs, Monkeys, Guinea pigs	Single or scattered lesions, circular with loss of hair, scaling and some erythema. Eczematous lesions reported	Bright yellow green fluorescence of infected hairs	Mycelium and chains of arthrospores	Sheath of small spores (2–3μ) in mosaic, completely surrounds hair at base. Easily dislodged from hair in preparation. Mycelium within hair running parallel to its length
Microsporum distortum	OCCASIONAL: Monkeys RARE: Dogs	Single or scattered lesions, circular with loss of hair and scaling	Bright yellow green fluorescence of infected hairs	Mycelium and chains of arthrospores	Same as above
Microsporum nanum	COMMON: Swine	Brown, crusty lesions (usually thin). Crusts may cover lesion uniformly, have a brown speckled appearance, or be more prominent at the periphery. Lesions may appear as urine or fecal stains. No pruritus or alopecia	No fluorescence	Branching mycelium	Large spores (5–8μ) in irregular chains on hair surface (human infections)
Microsporum vanbreuseghemii	RARE: Dogs, Squirrels	Circular, scaly lesions on dorsum and sides with alopecia	No fluorescence	Branching mycelium	Large spores in masses on hair surface
Microsporum cookei	RARE: Dogs, Cats, Baboons, Guinea pigs	Usually no lesions. Probable low order of pathogenicity. Diffuse, widespread alopecia and intense desquamation of inguinal region (baboon)	No fluorescence	Branching mycelium, few arthrospores	Endo-ectothrix hair invasion

* Adapted from Georg, L. K., *Animal Ringworm in Public Health*, Washington, U. S. Dept. of Health, Education and Welfare, 1959.

5

TABLE 1-1. (continued)

Fungus Species	Animals Affected	Location and Appearance of Lesions	Wood's Light Examination	Direct Examination in KOH Mounts	
				Skin Scrapings	Hair
		TRICHOPHYTON INFECTIONS			
Trichophyton mentagrophytes	COMMON: Dogs Cats Rabbits Chinchillas Guinea pigs Mice Rats	Most common on head near mouth and eyes, or at base of tail, but may be anywhere on body. Infection may be clinically inapparent. Usually irregularly defined areas of hair loss with considerable scaling are found. Heavy crusts may form. Occasionally pustules form at edges of lesion and suppuration beneath crusts	No fluorescence	Mycelium and chains of arthrospores	Sheath or isolated chains of spores $(3-5\mu)$ on surface of hair. Mycelium within hair
	OCCASIONAL: Horses Cows Muskrats Opposums Squirrels Foxes	Horse: lesions particularly in harness areas ("girth itch") Wild rodents: infections often clinically inapparent. In rodent epizootics, lesions may be heavy raised crusts of "favic type"			
	RARE: Swine				
Trichophyton verrucosum	COMMON: Cattle RARE: Horses Donkeys Burros Dogs Sheep	Usually on head or neck, but may be scattered on body, legs or tail. In calves lesions may be very extensive. Coin-sized or larger distinct plaques with heavy greyish white crusts. When crusts are removed, moist, bleeding areas are seen. Old lesions lose heavy crusts, show scaliness and broken-off hair stumps	No fluorescence	Mycelium and chains of arthrospores	Sheath or isolated chains of large spores $(5-10\mu)$ on surface of hair

Organism	Hosts	Lesions	Fluorescence	Mycelium	Hair
Trichophyton gallinae	COMMON: Chickens Turkeys RARE: Wild birds Dogs	White powdery scaliness which tends to form concentric rings on comb and wattles. Later heavy white crusts form in these areas ("white comb" or "favus of chickens"). In rare cases infection may spread over body which shows scaliness of the skin. Does not involve the feathers	No fluorescence	Mycelium and chains of arthrospores	Feathers not affected
Trichophyton equinum	COMMON: Horses RARE: Dogs	Scattered lesions especially in saddle area ("girth itch"). Circular lesions with matting of hair followed by hair loss and development of crusts. As lesions heal crusts fall off leaving bald areas and giving the animal a "moth-eaten" appearance	No fluorescence	Mycelium and chains of arthrospores	Sheath or isolated chains of spores ($3.5-8\mu$) on surface hair. Mycelium within hair
Trichophyton schoenleinii	OCCASIONAL: Dogs Cats Mice Monkeys	Commonly on the head, and occasionally on the back. Heavy yellowish crusts depressed at their centers to form "cups" or "scutula." Crusts may be agglomerated to form large masses. These are tightly adherent to the skin which bleeds when they are removed	Not reported in animals. (In human infections, none or dull whitish fluorescence has been reported)	Masses of very irregular mycelium and arthrospores some in chains	Hair invasion not reported in animals. In human infections, hairs are invaded throughout their length by branching mycelium which contain vacuoles and fat droplets
Trichophyton rubrum	RARE: Dogs Cows	Single or scattered lesions showing loss of hair, scaling and erythema	No fluorescence	Branching mycelium	Hair invasion rare. In experimental animal infections, chains of spores have been observed on outside of hair, and mycelium within hair
Trichophyton violaceum	RARE: Cows	Lesions similar to those caused by *T. verrucosum* in cattle	No fluorescence	Branching mycelium	Not reported in animals (endothrix in humans)
Trichophyton ajelloi	RARE: Horses	Scattered lesions with hair loss and scaling	No fluorescence	Mycelium and chains of arthrospores	Mycelium within hairs. No distinct sheath of spores about hairs

areas having hot and humid climatic conditions. There are interesting geographic differences with regard to the endemicity of the important dermatophytes. For example, *Microsporum canis* is the etiologic agent of approximately 98 percent of feline ringworm and 70 percent of canine ringworm cases in North America. In Czechoslovakia, where animal dermatomycosis is apparently quite common, this fungus has not been isolated.[12]

Due largely to the fact that it is not a reportable disease, the incidence of ringworm in animals is not precisely known. At the Small Animal Clinic of the University of Pennsylvania, a small segment of the total number of dermatologic presentations have fungal causes. In the more hot and humid southern climates, the incidence is considerably higher; in many areas along the Gulf Coast, particularly in summer, some clinicians diagnose the disease almost daily. In a colder climate, Pepin and Austwick culturally proved nearly one-fourth of 2368 cases of suspected ringworm.[13]

CLINICAL SIGNS AND PATHOLOGY

The pathogenesis of ringworm involving hairy skin has been studied extensively. Initially, it should be understood that when a dermatophyte contacts animal skin a number of events may occur. The fungus may be brushed off mechanically, it may not be able to establish residence primarily because of its inability to compete with the normal bacterial flora, it may establish residence on the skin but not produce a recognizable lesion, or finally it may establish residence on the skin and produce clinical disease. As was mentioned previously, the dermatophytes are not invasive organisms and their existence on the skin is limited to dead tissues, the keratin of the stratum corneum, hair and nail. Their primary direction of growth is downward rather than lateral; in order to survive, this growth must equal the normal desquamative process (the direction of which is outward).

As the dermatophyte does not invade living tissue, the only mechanism left by which the organism may produce disease is through the elaboration or excretion of toxins (irritants) or allergens. These substances find their way through the living epidermis into the dermal tissue where a vascular component is present and potentially capable of responding to the challenge of toxic or allergenic material through an inflammatory reaction. Thus, in a sense, ringworm is a biologic contact dermatitis.

In addition to the other challenges the dermatophyte faces to maintain itself on animal skin, the fungus' existence depends to a large degree on not evoking an inflammatory reaction. The dermatophytes have adapted through a long term evolutionary process to survive on a particular host skin (e.g. *Microsporum canis* on feline skin, *Trichophyton verrucosum* on bovine skin). Under ideal parasitic conditions, the fungi elaborate minimal or inadequate amounts of toxins or allergens to elicit an intense inflammatory reaction and thereby insure the inhabitation of its host's skin. It is known that when a zoophilic organism infects human skin a violent eruption occurs which may eliminate the infection. Similarly, an anthropophilic dermatophytic infection of animal skin is highly eruptive and may be short-lived.

As in other infectious disease processes, the lesion depends not only on the infectious agent but also upon the host's reactivity. In other words, a disease process with all its variables is the result of the interplay between the host and the infectious agent. When ringworm is a clinically recognizable disease, the dermatophyte has exceeded the limits of a balanced host-parasite relationship (elaborating toxins or allergens quantitatively or qualitatively capable of inducing inflammation), or the reactive threshold of the host has been reached.

When the dermatophyte causes a clinically recognizable disease, the following events occur. Through the production of toxins and allergens capable of evoking an inflammatory response by the host, the usual signs of an inflammatory reaction occur at the site of the infection—erythema, exudation, heat and alopecia. Since the dermatophyte usually is not capable of surviving an inflammatory reaction, it tends to move peripherally away from the inflammatory reaction and take up residence in adjacent normal tissue. The same inflammatory events which occurred originally follow in the new residence of the dermatophyte, and again the organism moves peripherally toward normal adjacent skin. This peripheral movement of the dermatophyte away from the inflammatory reaction creates the classical "ringed" lesion, which now appears as a circular patch of alopecia with central healing and an inflammatory reaction at the periphery. There comes a time when the expansive movement of the dermatophyte and the lesion terminates; after an unpredictable period of time the lesion becomes static, and the dermatophytic infection may end with self-healing.

The clinical manifestations of ringworm in domestic animals are extremely variable. The infinite variety of lesions relates to the interplay of the dermatophyte on one hand and the reactive capacity of the host on the other hand. At one end of the spectrum is the asymptomatic carrier and at the other extreme is a violently eruptive nodular or tumorous lesion referred to as a kerion (Fig. 1–1). The typical "ringed" lesion (Fig. 1–2) often is the exception rather than the rule. A clinical type of

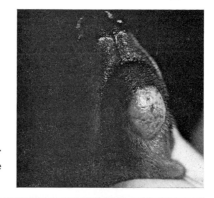

Fig. 1–1. Kerion reaction on chin of dachshund. The multiple follicular tracts can be seen.

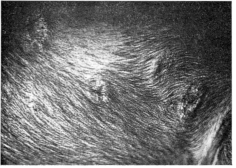

Fig. 1–2. Classical ringed or annular lesion of dermatophytosis. Note active border.

ringworm which is often misdiagnosed is the follicular papule or pustule from which staphylococcal organisms also may be cultured (Fig. 1–3). This lesion represents a mixed bacterial and dermatophytic infection.

The various species of animals exhibit a wide variation in the clinical signs of dermatomycosis. Review articles dealing with this subject may be found in the literature.[11,13,14] Table 1–1 is a listing of dermatophytic species which infect domestic animals. The following is a brief description of the most common infections and their clinical manifestations:

In cats and dogs, the most common causative dermatophyte is *Microsporum canis*. In the cat the lesions are usually found on the ears, face and extremities. Patches of alopecia with minimal erythema, or crusty alopecic patches are the typical lesions displayed (Figs. 1–4, 1–5). In dogs lesions usually occur on the face (particularly on the muzzle area), extremities and the lower abdomen; a crusty, alopecic eruption generally is representative (Fig. 1–6).

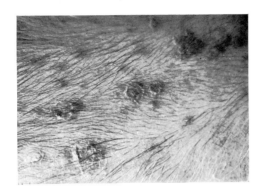

Fig. 1–3. Follicular pustules on groin resulting from a mixed dermatophytic and staphylococcal infection

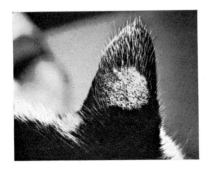

Fig. 1–4. A typical ringworm lesion on a cat. The crusty patch of alopecia on the pinna can be seen.

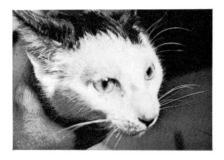

Fig. 1–5. Feline ringworm, with non-reactive alopecia lesion on face, medial and dorsal to left eye.

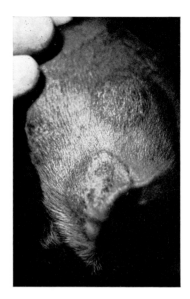

Fig. 1–6. Canine ringworm. Note active border and central clearing.

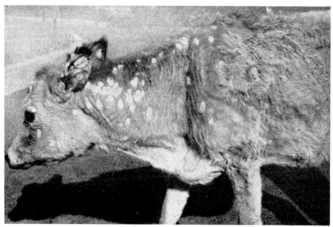

Fig. 1–7. Ringworm—caused by *Trichophyton verrucosum*. (Král and Schwartzman, Veterinary and Comparative Dermatology, courtesy of J. B. Lippincott Company)

Trichophyton verrucosum is the organism most frequently isolated from the lesions of cows. Eruptions occur commonly on the face and neck; a raised, crusty plaque or nodular lesion is characteristic of the infection (Fig. 1–7). Multiple (more than 10) lesions are usual.

In the horse, *Trichophyton equinum* and *Trichophyton mentagrophytes* are the most common etiologic agents. The region most frequently affected is the girth. Lesions vary from urticarial-like eruptions, patches of alopecia and scaling, to deep ulcerative nodules (Figs. 1–8, 1–9).

In sheep, species of the genus *Trichophyton* usually are causative though in general the disease is quite rare. The eruptions appear as crusty patches on the back, shoulders, neck and chest (Fig. 1–10).

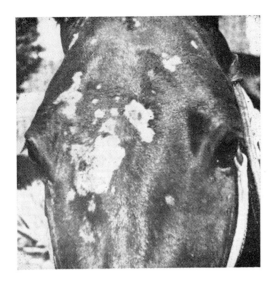

Fig. 1-8. Ringworm caused by *Trichophyton mentagrophytes.* (Král and Schwartzman, Veterinary and Comparative Dermatology, courtesy of J. B. Lippincott Company)

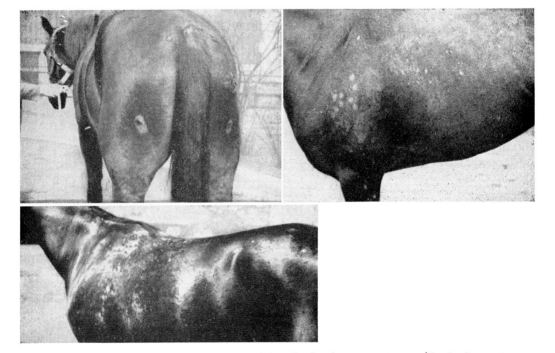

Fig. 1-9. Equine ringworm caused by *Trichophyton equinum.* (E. G. Batte in Král and Schwartzman, Veterinary and Comparative Dermatology, courtesy of J. B. Lippincott Company)

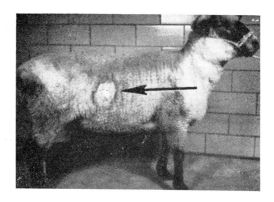

Fig. 1–10. Ringworm caused by *Trichophyton verrucosum.* (W. R. Pritchard in Král and Schwartzman, Veterinary and Comparative Dermatology, courtesy of J. B. Lippincott Company)

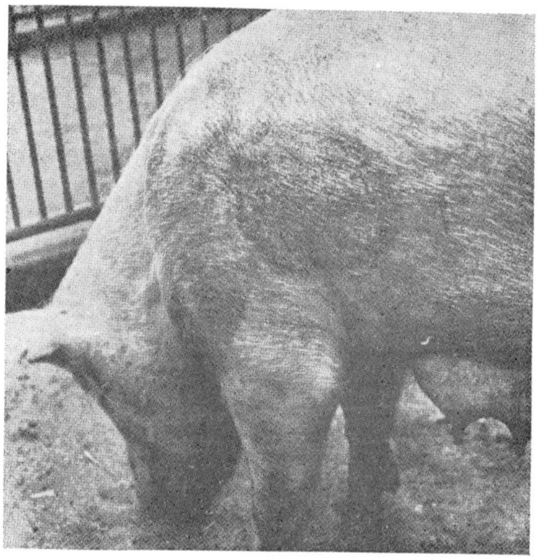

Fig. 1–11. *Microsporum nanum* lesion just caudal to the shoulder is red with a 2.5-cm. outer band of brown crusts giving it a ringworm appearance. (Ginther, Bubash and Ajello, *Microsporum nanum* infection in swine, courtesy of Veterinary Medicine/Small Animal Clinician)

Ringworm in goats is extremely rare. *Trichophyton* spp. are usually causative. Scaly and alopecic eruptions are the usual clinical manifestations of the disease and occur on the facial region and pinna.

In the pig, *Microsporum nanum* is usually the responsible dermatophyte. *Trichophyton* spp. have been identified in a few cases. Infections with *Microsporum nanum* produce lesions which occur primarily on the trunk (Fig. 1–11). They are slowly progressing, reddish brown, scaly or crusty discolorations of the skin which are difficult to recognize as hair loss is not a prominent feature of the disease.[15]

As in other infectious diseases, a definitive diagnosis of ringworm depends upon the demonstration of the causal agent. Diagnosis based on the clinical appearance of the lesion is difficult except in the exceptional classical "ringed" lesion. Other dermatoses such as bacterial infections, urticaria, seborrhea and tumors may be mistaken for a dermatophytic infection. The appearance of typical or atypical lesions in the areas mentioned for each animal host should suggest a possible diagnosis of ringworm and prompt the clinician to do further diagnostic procedures.

The diagnosis of ringworm on the basis of Wood's lamp examination of lesions is not always correct. A limited number of dermatophytes living on keratin produce a fluorescent yellow green material when exposed to ultraviolet light. Unfortunately, only *Microsporum canis, M. distortum* and *M. audouinii* are capable of producing this fluorescence in animals. Thus, the use of the Wood's lamp has limited diagnostic value and gives positive results only when infections by these organisms are involved. It is worth emphasizing also that nonfluorescing strains of *Microsporum canis* are encountered occasionally and that in an inflammatory lesion the infected hair stumps may be below the level of the skin surface and therefore fluorescence may not be seen. Thus, positive findings are significant but false negative findings are not unusual. Perhaps the most important utilization of the Wood's lamp is that of screening an asymptomatic carrier.* It is important to appreciate the fact that other materials, particularly medicaments (as salicylic acid), may fluoresce. The scale of dandruff will show itself under ultraviolet light with a dull (nonfluorescent) yellow color which should not be mistaken for the true yellowish green fluorescence of some dermatophytic infections.

The histopathologic features of ringworm are as variable as are the clinical manifestations of the disease. Little to no inflammatory reaction may be observed in association with the presence of spores and hyphae in the stratum corneum or on the hair shafts. On the other hand, an intense and destructive inflammatory reaction of the integument without evidence of fungal elements may be the major pathologic finding.

Microscopic examination of sections prepared from minimally inflamed but alopecic lesions reveals slight to moderate hyperkeratosis of the epidermis and follicles, acanthosis and a minimal perifollicular inflammatory reaction with a predominantly mononuclear cell infiltration. Fungal elements almost always may be visualized when sections are stained with silver methenamine or by the periodic acid-Schiff reaction. As the lesions become more inflammatory (ulceration, exudation, crusting), the surface epithelium may be observed to be in varying degrees of infiltration and destruction. Ulceration of the epidermis and replacement by an inflammatory crust is not uncommon. The walls of the infected hair follicles also are invaded by a dense inflammatory cell infiltration consisting of neutrophils, lymphocytes, histiocytes and plasma cells. This reaction may be so intense that no follicular structure is recognizable other than the hair shaft which lies free in the inflammatory reaction; the inflammatory reaction may show both granulomatous and abscessation patterns. As the inflammatory reaction destroys the dermatophytic infection, one usually cannot visualize fungal elements at this stage.

LABORATORY DIAGNOSIS

Direct Microscopic Examination

Microscopic examination of hair or scale is a rapid and reliable method of diagnosing ringworm. A small amount of hair and scale scraped from the periphery of the lesion should be placed in two or three drops of 10 per cent potassium hydroxide for 10 or 15 minutes before being cover-slipped. Gentle heating of the slide facilitates clearing of the material. Care should be taken not to place an excessive amount of hair or scale on the slide as it may impede visualizing the fungal elements.

* Another useful method of detecting an asymptomatic carrier is by employing the brush technique.[16] It consists essentially of running a clean or sterile toothbrush (small animals) or hand scrub brush (large animals) through the pelage in areas where lesions commonly occur. The brush bristles then are depressed in Sabouraud's medium and sufficient hair and scale deposited on the media for growth of fungus, if present, to occur. This method may be found useful also to collect material for culture from dry, scaly, alopecic lesions.

The material should be examined first under low magnification with the diaphragm partially closed to obtain visual contrast. Scanning the material, one should look for a hair which appears broken or deformed and then switch objectives to high magnification. Spores, rather than hyphae, are found most often in animal tissue being examined and usually they are concentrated in clusters (mosaic) or chains on the hair (Figs. 1–12, 1–13). Generally, the longer the material sits in the potassium hydroxide, the more accurate the examination. Allowing the slides to sit overnight in a humidifying chamber greatly facilitates viewing the spores.

The advantage of the direct microscopic method of diagnosis over other methods is that within a short time a definitive diagnosis can be made and therapy can be instituted with the initial examinition of the patient.

Culture

Diagnosing ringworm by cultural methods is the most reliable. Material (hair and scale) from the periphery of the lesion is taken as for microscopic examination and placed on a suitable culture medium. The collection site should be cleaned first with soap and water, then alcohol, to remove as completely as possible bacterial and fungal contaminants in the area. If fluorescing hairs are present, they should be collected while using a Wood's lamp.

Alopecic areas are examined carefully for stubby, broken hairs and, if found, are collected by pulling them from the follicle. Sterile or flamed scalpel and forceps should be used for collection. Collected material should be placed in a clean envelope rather than in an air-tight container especially if the material for culture is to be mailed or delayed.

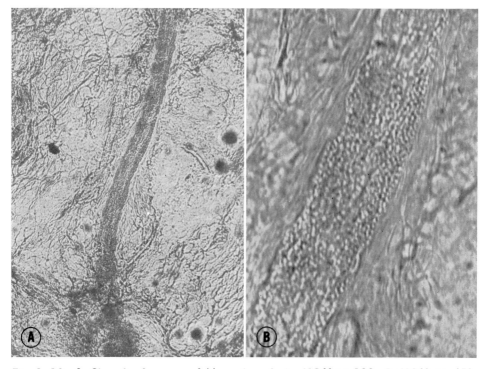

Fig. 1–12. **A.** Sheath of spores of M. *canis* on hair. KOH × 100. **B.** KOH × 450.

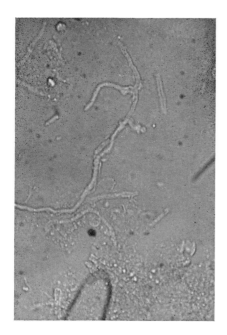

Fig. 1–13. Hyphae in skin scraping.
KOH × 450.

By means of aseptic techniques, the hairs and scale are placed on the surface of agar culture medium and pressed firmly into the agar. Many mycologists prefer agar slants in cotton plugged tubes to allow for an exchange of gases through the plug. This is necessary for both normal growth and pigment production. If screw-capped bottles or tubes are used, the caps should be slightly loosened. Use of Petri dishes is generally proscribed because massive numbers of spores may escape into the air when the lid is lifted. However, plates are sometimes used in studies of colony morphology. In this case, use of a protective hood is recommended.

Sabouraud's dextrose agar with chloramphenicol (Chloromycetin*) and cycloheximide (Acti-dione†) added is an excellent isolation medium. The acidity of Sabouraud's agar inhibits most bacteria. Chloramphenicol further restricts bacterial growth, and cycloheximide inhibits most saprophytic (contaminant) fungi. This medium is readily available from several sources under various trade names.

Vitamin enrichment of the media is necessary to grow certain dermatophytes. *Trichophyton equinum* requires nicotinic acid, and *Trichophyton verrucosum* requires thiamine and inositol. Also, *T. verrucosum* grows much faster at 37° C. than at room temperature.

Mycologists often inoculate tubes of Sabouraud-chloramphenicol-cycloheximide (Sabouraud C-C) agar and "plain" Sabouraud's dextrose agar in parallel. (Both are vitamin enriched if the material being cultured is from a cow or horse.) Pure colony isolations of dermatophytes are sometimes obtained on the "plain" Sabouraud agar, particularly if the lesion was carefully cleaned and most often if fluorescing hairs were selected. Colony growth is slightly faster on the less restrictive medium, and typical surface and reverse pigments may appear sooner. Also, some fungi usually considered to be contaminants occasionally cause lesions which

* Park, Davis & Company, Detroit, Michigan.
† The Upjohn Company, Kalamazoo, Michigan.

may be confused with ringworm (see Chapter 4). These will be restricted if Sabouraud C-C agar is used exclusively.

Culture tubes should be incubated at room temperature in a dark cabinet or drawer. The tubes should be held a minimum of 21 and preferably 30 days before discarding as negative. Identifiable growth of the dermatophytes often requires a minimum of five to eight days and sometimes requires longer incubation.

Gross colonial characteristics and pigmentation are helpful identification aids, but final identification requires microscopic study of the spores and their mycelial relationships. When working with fungus cultures, care must be used to prevent contaminating the worker and the surroundings. Aseptic techniques are used. It is advisable to place a paper towel over the work area of the table, and soak it with two percent Amphyl, pine oil, phenolic or some other disinfectant; this can then be folded and discarded upon completion of work.

For microscopic examination, a portion of the aerial growth is removed with a flamed, bent, bacteriologic inoculating needle or sterilized forceps and is placed in two or three drops of lacto phenol cotton blue stain on a clean glass slide. The matted mycelium may be gently teased apart with dissecting needles. The preparation is then gently cover-slipped before first low, then high power examination.

Because study of spore morphology and spore-mycelial relationships is necessary for fungal identification, mycologists often supplement their cultures with others grown by the slide culture method.

These are grown in a moist chamber prepared by placing a circular piece of filter paper in the bottom of a Petri dish. This is sterilized and a bent glass rod, well-flamed, is placed on the paper. Seven to eight mls. of sterile water or 10 percent glycerin in water is added aseptically. A flamed glass slide is then placed on top of the glass rod.

Cut a block of agar about 1 cm. square from a previously prepared agar plate. Using aseptic techniques throughout the procedure, transfer the agar block to the surface of the glass slide. Inoculate all four sides of the agar block with spores or mycelial growth of the fungus being studied. A flamed cover slip is then placed centrally over the agar block. Incubate in the dark until sporulation occurs. To examine, place a drop or two of lacto phenol cotton blue stain on a clean slide and gently place the cover slide on the stain.

Beautiful preparations result from this procedure with mycelium, spores and attachments intact. These mounts can be made semi-permanent by sealing the edges of the cover slide with nail polish.

Spore production has been stressed because of its importance in identifications. Occasionally an isolate sporulates poorly or not at all. In this case, transfers should be made to potato dextrose agar or rice grain medium.

Culture identification of dermatophytes is precise; unfortunately it is also slow. Therefore, the clinician and laboratorian should practice direct microscopic examination at every opportunity to become more proficient. Clinical judgment, skill with direct microscopic examinations, and cultures are all necessary for diagnostic excellence.

Until recently dermatophytes were classified as *Fungi Imperfecti* because only their asexual stage of reproduction was known. Discovery of the sexual stages of certain species of the genera *Microsporum* and *Trichophyton* now allows for a dual classification for the imperfect (*Microsporum* and *Trichophyton*) and perfect (*Nan-*

nizzia and *Arthroderma,* respectively) genera.[17]   A classification of dermatophytes may be made on various bases, but most simply by cultural and other differences related to certain morphologic characteristics, as conidia and other accessory structures.[18]   Two genera are of veterinary importance: *Microsporum* and *Trichophyton* (infections by species of the third genus, *Epidermophyton,* have not been described in domestic animals).

In general, the members of the genus *Microsporum* infect the hair and skin and usually form a mosaic sheath of arthrospores on or around the hair shafts.   In culture, they form cottony, wooly, matted or powdery colonies of various colors. Small (3–6μ), single-celled, clavate microconidia produced on short stalks or sessile on the hyphae are seen in microscopic mounts.   Large (8–15 × 40–150μ) multi-celled, thick- and rough-walled macroconidia are representative of the genus.   It is noteworthy that *Microsporum gypseum* and *M. nanum* have much thinner-walled macroconidia than other species in the genus.   The *Trichophyton* species infect skin, hair and nails; usually the arthrospores are arranged in parallel rows on or within the hair shafts.   In culture, granular to powdery, glabrous, smooth or waxy colonies with variable color are characteristic.   Numerous, small (2–4μ) microconidia and few large (4–6 × 10–50μ), multi-celled, smooth, thin-walled, clavate or pencil-shaped macroconidia may be visualized microscopically.   Coiled hyphae (spirals) are produced in many isolates, especially *T. mentagrophytes.*

Described below are the cultural and microscopic features of the more important dermatophytes infecting domestic animals.[2,18,19]   A more complete survey is presented in Table 1–2.

Microsporum canis (*M. felineum, M. equinum*).   Colonies grow rapidly and appear cottony, coarsely fluffy or woolly and eventually powdery with a light brown central area. On the reverse side, a bright yellow to orange coloration is characteristic. Numerous large (15–20 × 60–125μ), thick-walled (4μ), spindle-shaped, multiseptate (8–15 cells) macroconidia and a few small, single-celled, clavate microconidia, borne laterally along hyphae, may be seen in microscopic mounts.

Microsporum gypseum.   Colonies are flat and coarsely granular; a white and fluffy, sterile (pleomorphic) growth often appears in patches on the colony surface which is light brown to cinnamon brown in color.   The reverse color is pale yellow to tan.   Numerous large, four- to six-celled, ellipsoidal, rough-walled, thin-walled macroconidia and a few single-celled clavate microconidia are usually sessile on the hyphae.

Microsporum nanum.   Young colonies are white and cottony becoming granular and buff-colored with age; brown to red pigment appears on the reverse.   Abundant thin-walled, rough-walled, pear-shaped macroconidia with one or two septations are seen.

Trichophyton mentagrophytes (*Zoophilic Strain*).   Colonies are fast growing, coarsely granular or powdery with a white to cream to tan surface color and yellowish-rose to red on the reverse.   Macroconidia are usually scarce, club-shaped, thin-walled, smooth-walled and multiseptate; microconidia are quite numerous, single and in clusters (en grappe) along the hyphae.   Spirals are usually found.   Nodular bodies, chlamydospores and racquet hyphae may be seen.

Trichophyton equinum.   Young colonies are white and fluffy with brilliant yellow on the reverse (grossly resembles *M. canis*).   Older colonies become velvety and folded on surface and red-brown on the reverse.   Macroconidia are very rare with

TABLE 1–2.   Cultural Characteristics of Ringworm Fungi Isolated from Animals*

Fungus Species	Colony—Sabouraud Dextrose Agar with or without Antibiotics	Microscopic Characteristics
MICROSPORUM SPECIES		
Microsporum canis (Syn: M. lanosum, M. felineum M. equinum)	Growth rapid. Surface at first white, silky, with bright yellow pigment in peripheral growth. After two to four weeks, surface dense, tan, cottony, sometimes in irregular tufts or concentric rings, often with central knob of heavier growth. Reverse side of colony bright yellow, becomes dull orange brown. Rare strains show no pigment on reverse. Grows well on rice grains	Macroconidia numerous, 8–15 celled, spindle-shaped, often terminating in a distinct knob, and with thick, verrucose walls. Microconidia few, clavate, usually sessile on the hyphae
Microsporum gypseum (Syn: M. fulvum, Achorion gypseum)	Growth rapid. Colony flat with irregularly fringed border and coarsely powdery surface ranging from light ochre to deep cinnamon brown. Tufts of white, fluffy, sterile (pleo-morphic) growth develop rapidly on surface of colony, dull yellow to tan, rarely pinkish to red. Good growth on rice grains	Macroconidia numerous, 3–9 celled, ellipsoid, shorter and broader than those of M. canis and with thinner, rough walls. Microconidia rare, clavate, usually sessile on the hyphae
Microsporum audouinii	Colony slow growing, flat, velvety, with whitish tan to brownish surface. Reverse side of colony, light salmon, orange tan, or non-pigmented. Growth on rice grains very poor	Mycelium usually sterile with many chlamydospores. Microconidia usually rare, clavate, sessile on the hyphae. Macroconidia usually absent, but small numbers found in some strains. When present, are large, irregularly spindle-shaped, thick-walled with a smooth or rough surface. Abortive and bizarre-shaped macroconidia are most commonly seen
Microsporum distortum	Growth rapid. Colony flat with a tendency to develop radial grooves. Surface velvety to fluffy, white to tan. Some strains have little aerial mycelium and appear waxy. Reverse side of colony colorless to dull yellowish tan. Good growth on rice grains	Macroconidia numerous. They are thick-walled with a rough surface and markedly distorted in shape. Microconidia pear-shaped, sessile on the hyphae
Microsporum nanum	Growth rapid. Surface is at first white and cottony. Becomes granular and buff-colored with age. Brownish red on reverse	Macroconidia numerous, two- or three-celled, echinulate, pyriform and relatively thin-walled. Microconidia few to many, ovoid to clavate

* Adapted from Georg, L. K., Animal Ringworm in Public Health, Washington, U.S. Dept. of Health, Education and Welfare, 1959.

TABLE 1–2.   (Continued)

Fungus Species	Colony—Sabouraud Dextrose Agar with or without Antibiotics	Microscopic Characteristics
Microsporum vanbreuseghemii	Growth rapid. Surface growth flat, powdery to fluffy. Color white to light yellow or pink to deep rose. Reverse pigment lacking or light to lemon yellow	Macroconidia numerous, 5- to 12-celled, cylindro-fusiform, thick echinulate walls. Micro-conidia numerous, pyriform to obovate
Microsporum cookei	Growth rapid. Colony surface with powdery, yellow tan center, peripheral growth downy and white. Reverse pigment purplish red	Macroconidia numerous, multi-celled, elliptical, thick-walled and echinulate. Numerous hyaline, clavate microconidia borne singly

TRICHOPHYTON SPECIES

Fungus Species	Colony—Sabouraud Dextrose Agar with or without Antibiotics	Microscopic Characteristics
Trichophyton mentagrophytes (Syn: T. gypseum, T. granulosum, T. quinckeanum)	Growth rapid. Colony flat, or heaped and irregularly folded. Surface coarsely granular to powdery to downy, or cottony, white to cream, occasionally yellow or pink. Reverse side of colony, rose brown, occasionally yellowish, orange or deep red	Microconidia very numerous, small globose to slender and elongate borne singly along hyphae or in pine-tree-like terminal clusters. Macro-conidia rare or abundant in some strains, two- to five-celled, thin-walled, slightly club-shaped, spindle-shaped, or long and nearly pencil-shaped. Tightly wound spirals, nodular bodies may be numerous
Trichophyton verrucosum (Syn: T. faviforme, T. album, T. discoides, T. ochraceum)	Growth very slow, may not appear until 10 to 14 days incubation. Colony usually small, heaped and folded, occasionally flat and disc-shaped. Colonies at first glabrous and waxy, some-times developing white or yellow powdery or downy surface growth. No growth on vitamin-free media. Most strains require thiamine and inositol, some require thiamine only. Growth more rapid at 37° C.	On Sabouraud's dextrose agar, usually only a thin irregular mycelium with chlamydospores. If grown at 37° C., chlamydo-spores very numerous and form heavy chains. On thiamine-enriched media, mycelium is more regular and micro-conidia may be numerous. They are small and delicate borne singly along hyphae. Macroconidia extremely rare, three- to five-celled, thin, smooth walls, vary considerably in size and shape
Trichophyton equinum	Growth rapid. Colony flat, but develops folds with age. Surface at first white and fluffy with bright yellow pigment in peripheral growth. Later surface becomes flatter and velvety and cream to tan. Reverse side of colony at first bright yellow, later pink to deep red brown. No growth on vitamin-free media. All strains require nicotinic acid	Microconidia few to many. Generally thin and elongate. Macroconidia very rare with thin, smooth walls

TABLE 1–2.   (Continued)

Fungus Species	Colony—Sabouraud Dextrose Agar with or without Antibiotics	Microscopic Characteristics
Trichophyton schoenleinii (Syn: *Achorion schoenleinii*)	Growth slow, usually irregularly heaped and folded, tough and leathery, tending to crack the agar. Surface white to tan, glabrous and waxy or white with powdery or downy surface growth. Occasional strains grow largely submerged in the agar. All strains will grow in a vitamin-free medium. Grows as well at room temperature as at 37° C.	Mycelium highly irregular. Coarser hyphae tend to become knobby and clubbed at ends (chandeliers). Chlamydospores usually numerous. Microconidia very rare. Macroconidia absent
Trichophyton rubrum (Syn: *T. purpureum*)	Growth slow. Colony flat or heaped, with a white fluffy surface. Occasional strains with a powdery or velvety surface which becomes highly folded. Such strains are at first white to cream in color, but later become a deep rose. Reverse side of most isolates shows a red to deep purplish red pigmentation. This disappears in subcultures. Rare strains lack this deep red pigment on first isolation, may be yellowish orange on reverse	Microconidia rare in most fluffy strains, thin and delicate and occurring only along sides of hyphae. Microconidia common in velvety or granular strains, more globose and occurring along the mycelium and in pine-tree-like clusters. Macroconidia rare in most strains, but most common in granular cultures, usually elongate and thin with parallel sides and blunt ends, three to eight cells
Trichophyton violaceum	Growth very slow. Colony heaped and verrucose. Surface glabrous, at first cream then lavender becoming deep purple. Old cultures may develop downy surface growth, may lose purple pigment	Mycelium thin, irregular with chlamydospores. Microconidia usually not found
Trichophyton ajelloi	Growth rapid. Colony flat or somewhat heaped and folded. Surface finely powdery or downy, cream to tan or orange tan in color. Areas of white fluffy (pleomorphic) growth develop rapidly. Reverse side of colony is colorless or a deep bluish black	Macroconidia numerous. They are long and slender with parallel walls tapering at each end (cylindrofusiform) and composed of 8 to 12 cells. The walls of macroconidia are wide (thicker than those of M. canis) and have a smooth surface. Microconidia abundant in some strains, rare in others, ovate to pyriform sessile on the hyphae
Trichophyton gallinae (Syn: *Achorion gallinae*)	Growth rapid. Colony surface flat with irregular folds, downy to fluffy. Color white to pink. Reverse pigment strawberry red. Medium becomes deep red from diffusion of pigment	Macroconidia numerous, 2- to 10-celled, large with smooth double-contoured walls. Single-celled microconidia rare

thin, smooth walls. Microconidia vary from few to many and are thin and elongate. No growth occurs on vitamin-free media; nicotinic acid is required for growth.

Trichophyton verrucosum. Colonies are slow growing and require vitamin enrichment (thiamine and inositol). They are raised, glabrous and yellowish or greyish. Finally, they develop scant aerial growth. Old colonies are very tough (rubbery). There are antlerlike branching hyphae (on Sabouraud's agar) and chlamydospores often in chains. Macroconidia are very rare and few microconidia appear on vitamin-enriched media. Growth is more rapid at 37° C.

Pathogenicity Tests

Production of an infection in the integument of laboratory animals with hair or scale from a ringworm lesion of a patient is easily achieved but of no practical importance. Interestingly, the infections usually terminate spontaneously in three or four weeks.

Immunology

It is well-established that the tissues contain a "serum factor" which is fungistatic or fungicidal in its effect and apparently restricts dermatophytes to keratinized tissues. Attempts to define this factor (in particular, to identify it as an antibody) have not been successful. However, the factor is present at birth and does not vary significantly with age.[20] Until recently, attempts to demonstrate antibodies against dermatophytes have generally been unrewarding. Reyes and Friedman[21] have shown unequivocally that dermatophyte mycelia are capable of stimulating good antibody response in experimental animals. McNall and associates[22] have studied the antigenic fraction of the outer wall of *Trichophyton mentagrophytes* and shown it to be a polysaccharide. It is highly antigenic and induces the production of appreciable quantities of antibodies. Both groups of investigators report on cross reactions between various dermatophytes and common fungal contaminants.

Though the dermatophytes appear to be of low antigenicity, they are highly allergic. Hypersensitivity reactions are a common phenomenon associated with dermatophytic infections. In the dog, the intradermal injection of microsporin (following an infection by *Microsporum canis*) evokes a 24- to 48-hour papular reaction. Further evidence of a hypersensitivity phenomenon comes from the following observations:[23] under experimental conditions, if one infects a dog with *Microsporum canis*, the initial appearance of the lesion occurs two or three days after the occlusive dressing containing the dermatophyte is removed. The infection lasts for approximately 20 days, at which time no dermatophyte can be demonstrated. Complete healing with regrowth hair occurs one to four weeks following the termination of the dermatophytic infection. If within the next one to three months an attempt is made to infect the animal for a second time, the lesion which is produced differs in two ways: (1) it is of a more intense inflammatory nature; and (2) the dermatophyte can be demonstrated for only two or three days after the eruption becomes evident. The identical hypersensitivity phenomenon which is associated with an active infection can be produced experimentally by multiple intradermal injections of the extract of the dermatophyte—twice-weekly injections of microsporin are given for four weeks to produce a similar situation. Following experimental induction of the hypersensitivity, the application of a dermatophyte under an occlusive dressing produces a short-lived infection similar to a second infection in the same individual.   Florian and partners also have immunized calves against ringworm with a vaccine prepared from *Trichophyton verrucosum.*[24]

Though hypersensitivity often is an injurious and destructive phenomenon, in the case of a dermatophytic infection, it results in a protective mechanism which induces an inflammatory reaction of enough intensity to limit or terminate the infection.

DIFFERENTIAL DIAGNOSIS

In general, ringworm is overdiagnosed in veterinary medicine.   Such lesions as insect bites, urticaria, bacterial infections, seborrheic dermatitis and interdigital dermatitis often are confused with ringworm.   There is a temptation to diagnose a fungal infection on observing a circular or oval scaling lesion or when presented with an ill-defined pruritic dermatosis.   It is worth emphasizing that the skin usually reacts in a circular or oval pattern to the vast majority of insults which induce an inflammatory reaction.   Also, the diagnosis of ringworm on a clinical basis is fraught with error and can be made only upon demonstration of the dermatophyte by microscopic examination of tissue and/or by cultural methods.

EPIDEMIOLOGY

Ringworm is a zoonotic disease and, for both moral and legal reasons, the client should be advised of the possibility of infection for him or his family members.   In the authors' experience, most cases of animal ringworm involve the patient only and spare the family members.   However, zoophilic dermatophytes may cause human epidemics[9] and Kaplan and co-workers[25] reported that of 368 dogs with ringworm, ten percent of owner family members were infected also.   Thirty percent of owner family members with cats having ringworm were infected.   It should be noted that wild animals also contribute to the animal reservoir of ringworm.[26,27]

Though the usual route of infection is by direct contact, indirect contact and airborne infections also account for transmission of the disease.   Spores remain viable for months to years under normal environmental conditions.   The significance of these viable spores and the asymptomatic animal carrier has not been assessed fully in terms of their potential danger to man.

In urban areas, it is estimated that approximately 20 percent of human infections are of animal origin.   Children are involved more often and the scalp tends to be the most common site of the disease.   In rural areas, approximately 80 percent of human ringworm is of animal origin. The adult, rather than the child, is involved more often and the arms and face are the usual sites of eruption.

Ringworm is an important disease of domestic animals, particularly farm animals, in that it is: (1) potentially contagious and thus may affect a herd or group of animals; (2) may have a protracted course; (3) the dermatophytic spores remain viable in the environment for years and thus new animals brought into the area may be infected; (4) cross infections from animal to man may occur; (5) the disease may be pruritic and thus the animal suffers varying degrees of discomfort from the infection; and (6) though an animal may clinically recover from an infection, the dermatophytes may maintain residence on his skin or pelage, thus resulting in the establishment of an asymptomatic carrier state.

In general, young animals appear to be infected more often than adults.   There appears to be no sex or breed predilection but certain individuals or members of a particular family or breeding may be genetically predisposed.   In a number of instances, it has been observed that in catteries, certain animals and their progeny repeatedly are affected; whereas within this same environment, other animals with adequate exposure to infected cats do not develop the disease. Seasonal patterns of ringworm have been reported, e.g. the winter occurrence in cattle and horses (September through January).[13] Pet animals, particularly cats, often develop the disease shortly after weaning their litter.

There are a number of common misconceptions regarding ringworm. First, it is thought that ringworm is a highly contagious disease and that any individual exposed to an infected animal will develop the disease. This is not true. In many cases, cross infections from animals to another animal or to man do not occur, and it is tempting to generalize that ringworm is not highly contagious. However, this must also be qualified, because occasionally animal dermatophytic infections are quite contagious. It also is thought that ringworm in animals is a chronic progressive type of disease (as it may occur as a scalp infection in man). Though in some instances it does manifest itself in this manner, the disease in general is self-limiting and spontaneous recovery is common. This may relate to the shorter hair cycle in animals than in man. Another aspect of the disease which is not considered commonly is the viability of the spores. It is now abundantly clear that spores shed from an infected animal may remain viable and infectious for months to years under ordinary environmental conditions. The route of infection is most often by direct contact. Though this is perhaps the most common mechanism of infection, the disease may be transmitted also by the airborne route.[28] Finally, it often is considered that with clinical cure the dermatophyte no longer exists on the tissues of the host. Again this is not true because, as mentioned previously, the organism may continue to reside on the tissues of the animal after clinical recovery. Though no figures on the actual asymptomatic carrier rate of animals are available, it has been suggested that approximately 10 percent of cats are carrying *Microsporum canis* on their skin or pelage. Dogs also have been reported to carry dermatophytes asymptomatically.[29,30,31]

TREATMENT OF DERMATOPHYTOSES (RINGWORM)

The natural mechanisms which abort a dermatophytic infection should be emphasized before the drugs commonly employed in the treatment of the disease are discussed. Two reactions are involved in terminating an infection:[32] (1) the spontaneous or induced transformation of an anagen to a telogen stage (resting) hair; (2) the arrest of keratin production as a result of the effects of an intense inflammatory reaction on the hair bulb matrix. Both natural mechanisms have not received the credit which they deserve in resolving an infection which is often credited to the drug employed by the clinician.

Literally hundreds of topical agents are used in the treatment of ringworm. It must be understood that a significant difference exists in the therapeutic results obtained in employing topical agents to glabrous (non-hairy) skin and to hairy skin. Many topical agents are effective in the treatment of ringworm of glabrous skin but few if any are successful in managing ringworm of the scalp or hairy skin of animals. Since ringworm is often a self-limiting infection, the efficacy of any drug in the treatment of hairy skin must be proven with adequate controls.

It was not until the discovery and use of griseofulvin that a truly effective medicament for the treatment of ringworm of the hairy skin was realized. Griseofulvin is an antibiotic (a metabolic product of *Penicillium griseofulvin* Diercki) with specific activity against dermatophytes, but without activity against bacteria, yeasts and other fungi. The efficacy of the drug is well-established; reports dealing with the beneficial effects achieved in the treatment of ringworm in man and animals are abundant in the literature.[33,34,35,36,37] The action of the drug is primarily fungistatic; it impairs the development of the terminal hyphae and causes curling, thickening and distortion.[38] A fungicidal activity has been demonstrated with young actively growing fungal cells.[39,40] The susceptibility of dermatophytes to griseofulvin is variable and resistant strains have been reported.[41,42]

The drug has been prepared in two forms: for topical and oral administration. Results with topical therapy have been poor and the oral route of administration is accepted as the method of choice. When given per os, griseofulvin is absorbed poorly from the intestinal tract, but significant levels are present in the skin within one to four hours. Studies conducted in the dog and guinea pig indicated that it was excreted slowly as detectable levels were observed for seven days after the last dose was administered.[43] Increased absorption and higher blood levels of griseofulvin have been achieved with the use of the microcrystalline form of the drug.[44] In addition, absorption is facilitated by administering the drug with a meal high in fat content.

A variety of dose schedules are employed in practice: a single massive dose, once weekly, and daily administration. The authors prefer the daily administration of the drug (in microcrystalline form) at a dose rate of 10–20 mg./lb. with concomitant use of a topical agent. At the Veterinary Clinic of the University of Pennsylvania, the best therapeutic results have been achieved with griseofulvin and the topical application of Captan,* as a 1:200 solution applied every four days for six treatments. In general, griseofulvin is administered for one month; but the duration of treatment depends on clinical results and specifically on demonstrating the absence of the dermatophyte in the healed lesion. Higher dose rates and prolonged therapeutic programs occasionally may be necessary to achieve total elimination of the organism.

There are five classes in which agents used in the treatment of ringworm can be placed: (1) irritants, which by evoking an inflammatory reaction act against the infection; (2) keratolytics, which peel or remove the stratum corneum in which the dermatophytes reside; (3) fungicidal agents, which directly kill or destroy the dermatophyte; (4) fungistatic agents, which inhibit the growth of the dermatophyte; and (5) agents which convert anagen (actively growing) hairs to telogen (resting) hairs or which arrest keratin production—such as thallium or x-ray irradiation. Within these classes there are a vast number of topical agents presently employed in the treatment of ringworm. One hundred are listed in the *Physicians' Desk Reference;*[45] in addition, a conservative estimate of 20 products are sold under a veterinary label. It is obvious that a definitive topical agent is not available and that the use of any one agent is a matter of personal choice. As indicated previously, Captan is the authors' agent of choice as it has proven effective and economical. Solutions of fatty acids, as Sopronal† and Naprylate‡ also are employed commonly in our practice, particularly for cats or when lesions are limited.

* Orthocide Garden Fungicide, 50% Captan, Chevron Chemical Co., Ortho Division, San Francisco, California.
† Wyeth Laboratories, Philadelphia, Pennsylvania.
‡ Strasenburgh, Rochester, New York.

As in any dermatologic condition, the vehicular form of the medical treatment is dependent upon the morphologic features of the eruption. The acute eruption (weeping, erythematous, hot) should be treated most conservatively, and agents which might further irritate an already inflamed lesion should be avoided. Bland wet soaks are most applicable to the acute eruption and boric acid (two to five percent) or potassium permanganate (1:5000) are employed commonly. Chronic lesions (thickened skin, hyperpigmentation, crusting) and, in general, lesions in hairy areas are best treated with water soluble or miscible ointments (as carbowax or hydrophilic ointment) in which fungistatic or fungicidal agents have been incorporated. The use of lotions should be restricted to the treatment of subacute eruptions of the non-hairy skin.

Many of the products employed presently in the topical treatment of ringworm contain time-honored agents, either singly or in combination with one another: *precipitated sulfur* in concentrations of one to ten percent is fungicidal, may be incorporated into a variety of vehicles, and its antifungal activity probably relates to hydrogen sulfide, a reduction product of sulfur; *salicylic acid* is both keratolytic, antifungal and moderately irritating; concentrations from two to ten percent are employed; *fatty acids* as undecylenic, caprylic and proprionic are both fungistatic and fungicidal, non-irritating, extremely low in toxicity and uniformly effective against the broad spectrum of dermatophytes; *benzoic acid* in concentrations of six percent is antifungal, non-irritating and non-toxic; *resorcinol* may be employed in concentrations of one to ten percent and possesses antifungal and keratolytic activity; *phenol* is an antifungal agent which also is potentially irritating and toxic (systemically); it should be used in concentration of less than one percent; *iodine* is strongly fungicidal but because of its potential irritating effect should not be used in inflamed lesions; solutions and tinctures containing concentrations of two to five percent are recommended; *hydroxyquinolines*, in addition to being antieczematous and antibacterial, possess antifungal activity in concentrations of one to three percent. They commonly are marketed in an ointment form.

A number of antiseptic preparations with antifungal activity are available for treating instruments, cages, examination tables, stables, etc.: Wescodyne* and cresylic disinfectant are employed in our clinic.

In the practice of small animal medicine, it is advisable not to hospitalize an animal for the treatment of ringworm. Viable spores have been isolated from the air,[46] and airborne infections occur. Also, other patients and employees may become infected. Therefore, home treatment rather than hospitalization is recommended. The client should be advised to isolate the animal in an area in his home which can be sanitized, is out of the usual traffic pattern and in particular is an area from which children can be asked not to enter (as the garage, basement or breezeway). Only adults should be allowed to treat the patient and following treatment they should wash their hands or wear inexpensive disposable plastic gloves while treating the animal. The patient should be reexamined in two weeks, preferably not in the examination room or office but rather in the owner's car. Four weeks after the original visit the site should be reexamined for viable dermatophytes.

In the treatment of large animals, those infected should be kept and treated in the already contaminated area. Every effort should be made to destroy contaminated bedding and to disinfect equipment and objects in the environment with which the

* Interstate Chemical Company, Div. of West Chemical Products Inc., Kansas City, Missouri.

patients may have come in contact. New animals should not be brought into the area and similar instructions regarding personal care of the adult who is treating the patients should be given to the client. Topical applications of Captan have proven effective and economical for the treatment of ringworm in large animals as well. In rare instances, griseofulvin may have to be administered in conjunction with topical therapy.

REFERENCES

1. Weary, P. E. and Canby, C. M.: Keratolytic Activity of Trichophyton Schoenleini, Trichophyton Rubrum and Trichophyton Mentagrophytes. J. Invest. Derm., *48* (1967): 240–248.
2. Emmons, C. W., Binford, C. H., and Utz, J. P.: *Medical Mycology.* 2nd edition, Philadelphia, Lea & Febiger, 1970.
3. Megnin, P.: Nouvelle Maladie Parasitaire de la Peau Chez un Coq. Compt. Rend. Soc. Biol., *33* (1881): 404–406.
4. Sabouraud, R.: *Les Trichophyties Humaines.* Paris, Rueff et Cie, 1894.
5. Bodin, E.: *Les Teignes Tondantes du Cheval et Leurs Inoculations Humaines.* Paris, Thèse, 1896.
6. Bodin, E. and Almy, J.: Le Microsporum du Chien. Rec. Med. Vet., *VIII*(4), (1897): 161–183.
7. Matruchot, L. and Dassonville, C.: Sur un Nouveau Trichophyton Produisant L'herpes Chez le Cheval. Compt. Rend. Acad. Sci., Paris, *127* (1898): 279–281.
8. Sabouraud, R.: *Les Teignes.* Paris, Musson et Cie, 1910.
9. Blank, F.: Dermatophytes of Animal Origin Transmissible to Man. Amer. J. Med. Sci., *229* (1955): 302–316.
10. Georg, L. K.: *Animal Ringworm in Public Health.* Washington, D.C., U.S. Dept. of Health, Education and Welfare, 1959.
11. Dawson, C. O.: Ringworm in Animals. Rev. Med. Vet. Mycol., *6* (1968): 223–233.
12. Dvořák, J. and Otčenášek, M.: *Mycological Diagnosis of Animal Dermatophytoses.* The Hague, Dr. W. Junk N. V., Publishers, 1969.
13. Pepin, G. A. and Austwick, P. K. C.: Skin Diseases of Domestic Animals II.—Skin Disease, Mycological Origin. Vet. Rec., *82* (1968): 208–214.
14. Král, F. and Schwartzman, R. M.: *Veterinary and Comparative Dermatology.* Philadelphia, J. B. Lippincott Company, 1964.
15. Ginther, O. J.: Clinical Aspects of Microsporum Nanum Infections in Swine. J. Amer. Vet. Med. Ass., *146* (1965): 945–953.
16. Goldberg, H. C.: Brush Technique for Detection of Fungus Disease. J. Amer. Vet. Med. Ass., *147* (1965): 845.
17. Ajello, L.: A Taxonomic Review of the Dermatophytes and Related Species. Sabouraudia, *6* (1968): 147–159.
18. Conant, N. F., Smith, D. T., Baker, R. D., Callaway, J. L., and Martin, D. S.: *Manual of Clinical Mycology.* 2nd edition, Philadelphia, W. B. Saunders Co., 1954.
19. Rebell, G., Taplin, D., and Blank, H.: *Dermatophytes, Their Recognition and Identification.* Miami, Dermatology Foundation of Miami, 1964.
20. Lorincz, A. L., Priestly, J. O., and Jacobs, P. H.: Evidence of Humoral Mechanisms Which Prevents Growth of Dermatophytes. J. Invest. Derm., *31* (1958): 15–17.
21. Reyes, A. C. and Friedman, L.: Concerning the Specificity of Dermatophyte-Reacting Antibody in Human and Experimental Animal Sera. J. Invest. Derm., *47* (1966): 27–34.
22. McNall, E. G., Sternberg, T. H., Newcomer, V. D., and Sorenson, L. J.: Chemical and Immunological Studies on Dermatophyte Cell Wall Polysaccharides. J. Invest. Derm., *36* (1961): 155–157.
23. Schwartzman, R. M.: Unpublished data (1967).
24. Florian, E., Nemeseri, L., and Loůas, G.: Active Immunization of Calves Against Ringworm. Magy. Allatorv. Lap., *19* (1964): 529–530.
25. Kaplan, W., Georg, L. K., and Ajello, L.: Recent Developments in Animal Ringworm and Their Public Health Implications. Ann. N.Y. Acad. Sci., *70* (1958): 636–649.

26. McKeever, S., Menges, R. W., Kaplan, W., and Ajello, L.:   Ringworm Fungi of Feral Rodents in Southwestern Georgia. Amer. J. Vet. Res., *19* (1958): 969–972.
27. McKeever, S., Kaplan, W., and Ajello, L.:   Ringworm Fungi in Large Wild Mammals in Southwestern Georgia and Northwestern Florida. Amer. J. Vet. Res., *19* (1958): 973–975.
28. Uscavage, J. P. and Král, F.:   Microsporum Canis: Isolation from the Air. J. Small Anim. Pract., *1* (1961): 279–280.
29. Gip, L. and Martin, B.:   Isolation of Trichophyton Terrestre, Trichophyton Mentagrophytes Var. Asteroides and Trichophyton Rubrum from Dogs. Acta Dermatovener., *44* (1964): 248–250.
30. Gentles, J. C., Dawson, C. O., and Connole, M.D.:   Keratophilic Fungi on Cats and Dogs. Sabouraudia, *4* (1965): 171–175.
31. Connole, M. D.:   Keratophilic Fungi on Cats and Dogs. Sabouraudia, *4* (1965): 45–48.
32. Kligman, A. M.:   Tinea Capitis Due to M. Audiouini and M. Canis. Arch. Derm., *71* (1955): 313–337.
33. Blank, H. and Roth, F. J., Jr.:   The Treatment of Dermatomycoses with Orally Administered Griseofulvin. Arch. Derm., *79* (1959): 259–267.
34. Williams, D. I., Masten, R. H., and Sarkany, I.:   Oral Treatment of Ringworm with Griseofulvin. Lancet, *2* (1958): 1212–1213.
35. Kaplan, W. and Ajello, L.:   Therapy of Spontaneous Ringworm in Cats with Orally Administered Griseofulvin. Arch. Derm., *81* (1960): 714–723.
36. Lauder, I. M. and O'Sullivan, J. G.:   Ringworm in Cattle: Prevention and Treatment with Griseofulvin. Vet. Rec., *70* (1958): 949–951.
37. Uvarov, O.:   Veterinary Experience with Griseofulvin. Tr. St. John's Hosp. Derm. Soc., *45* (1960): 28.
38. Brian, P. W.:   Studies on the Biological Activity of Griseofulvin. Ann. Botany, London, *13* (1949): 59.
39. Foley, E. J. and Greco, G. A.:   Studies on the Mode of Action of Griseofulvin. *Antibiotics Annual.* New York, Medical Encyclopedia Inc., 1959–1960.
40. Blank, H. and Taplin, D.:   Electron Microscopic Observations of the Effects of Griseofulvin on Dermatophytes. Arch. Derm., *81* (1960): 667–680.
41. Gentles, J. C.:   Effects of Griseofulvin on Experimental Infections (1). Tr. St. John's Hosp. Derm. Soc., *45* (1960): 10.
42. Michaelides, P., Rosenthal, S. A., and Sulzberger, M. B.:   Trichophyton Tonsurans Infection Resistant to Griseofulvin. Arch. Derm., *83* (1961): 988–990.
43. Greco, G. A., Moss, E. L., and Foley, E. J.:   Observation on Treatment of Fungus Infections of Animals with Griseofulvin. *Antibiotics Annual.* New York, Medical Encyclopedia Inc., 1959–1960.
44. Crounse, R. J.:   Effective Use of Griseofulvin. Arch. Derm., *87* (1963): 176–178.
45. Miller, A. B., et al.: *Physicians' Desk Reference.* Oradell, N. J., Litton Publications, Inc., 1969.
46. Uscavage, J. P. and Král, F.:   Microsporum Canis: Isolation from the Air. J. Small Anim. Pract., *1* (1961): 279–280.

Part II

THE SUBCUTANEOUS AND INTERMEDIATE MYCOSES

CHAPTER 2 | Sporotrichosis

Sporotrichosis is a chronic granulomatous and usually subcutaneous infection caused by *Sporotrichum schenckii*. The disease has been reported in horses, mules, dogs, cats, cattle, camels, fowl, swine, rats, mice, hamsters, chimpanzees[2] and man.

HISTORY, GEOGRAPHIC DISTRIBUTION AND PREVALENCE

The first reported case of sporotrichosis in the United States was made by Schenck in 1899.[3] It was not until the early part of the twentieth century, however, that reports dealing with sporotrichosis in animals appeared in the literature.[4] The rat has the dubious honor of being the first animal species reported to be infected spontaneously. One year later, in 1908, a natural infection was reported in a dog, and in 1909, in horses and mules. Infections of other animal species were reported in the 1940s: camels,[5] domestic fowl[6] and cattle.[7] Within the last twenty years, most reports of sporotrichosis in domestic animals have dealt with the infection in horses,[8,9] dogs[10] and swine.[1]

The geographic distribution of sporotrichosis in animals is probably universal. However, reports have come only from the following countries: Brazil, Canada, Colombia, France, Greece, Indo-China, Italy, Madagascar (Malagasy Republic), South Africa, Syria and the United States. In these countries, the disease is usually endemic and rarely epidemic. In the United States, there may be a geographic prevalence of the human disease in the north central part of the country.

It is impossible to estimate the incidence of sporotrichosis in animals. The disease is not reportable, and thus data is not available for establishing this figure. A judgment based on the reports in the literature would be entirely fallacious as it depends upon the willingness of the clinician to report the disease, clinical acuity and diagnostic confirmation. As the organism is a ubiquitous saprophyte in nature, domestic animals and man have a known exposure potential. Sporotrichosis is primarily a wound infection, i.e., the organism is implanted into the subcutaneous tissue following injury to the skin. Thus all the variables associated with such an event in addition to the host-organism interplay are factors in determining whether an infection occurs.

CLINICAL SIGNS AND PATHOLOGY

Sporotrichosis occurs in two forms: an infection limited to the subcutaneous tissues and lymphatics, or a disseminated form in which, following the primary skin infection, metastatic lesions develop in internal organs. The vast majority of case reports dealing with the disease in animals indicate that the subcutaneous-lymphatic infection is characteristic of the animal disease. The disseminated form has been reported only in the dog.[11] Though species variations occur, the classical lesion of sporotrichosis in domestic animals is a subcutaneous nodule which may be ulcerative and/or suppurative.

In the horse, the infection appears to remain localized in the subcutaneous tissues. Two forms of the disease have been characterized: (1) an ulcerative lymphangitis in which nodules and later ulcers develop along lymph vessels, and (2) a subcutaneous form (without involvement of the lymphatic system) in which multiple nodules develop in the integumentary system and eventually ulcerate and drain.[12] Lesions invariably develop on the extremities, particularly the fetlock region.[13] A non-tender nodule(s) develops at the infection site and usually breaks down to form an ulcer which discharges a purulent exudate (Fig. 2–1). The initial lesion often heals in three or four weeks, only to be followed by the appearance of satellite lesions in the immediate area and along lymphatic channels. The latter development leads to a cording effect which is characteristic of the disease. Systemic signs are rare.[14] Davis and Worthington[8] reported on an unusual case of equine sporotrichosis in which the disease appeared to be manifested initially by acute central nervous system signs, including incoordination, falling backward and inability to stand. Three months following these initial signs, the animal developed lymphangitis of the left hind limb characterized by ulcerative nodules. As in man, dissemination of the infection from cutaneous sites is rare in the horse. Whether this relates to the low virulence of the organism, the development of immunity

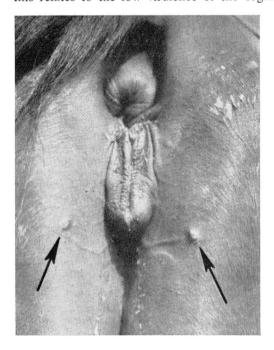

Fig. 2–1. Sporotrichosis in the beginning stage. (Král and Schwartzman, Veterinary and Comparative Dermatology, courtesy of J. B. Lippincott Company)

which counters the rapid spread of the organism (inadequate though to cure the disease), or to other factors is a moot point.

In the dog, both cutaneous and disseminated forms have been reported.[11,14] The more frequent involvement of internal organs in the dog contrasts with the infection in the equine species. The lymphangitic form, which is so typical of equine infections, has also been described in the dog.[14] Nodules develop along lymphatic vessels, appearing firm and tender to the touch, and eventually break down to form

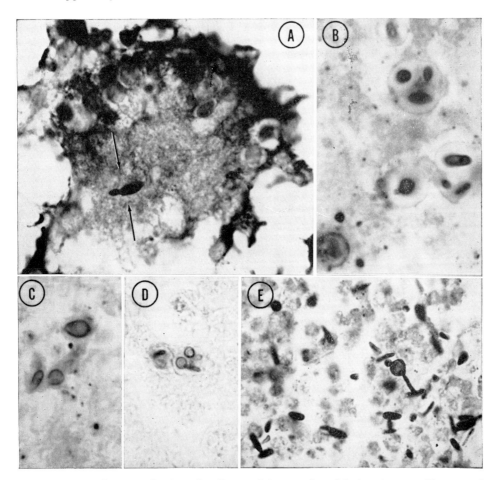

Fig. 2-2. Sporotrichosis. **A.** *Sporotrichum schenckii* in tissue. Elongated budding form in giant cell within a localized skin lesion, case from South Africa. PAS. × 1250. 1222221. (62–538). **B.** Meningeal abscess containing *S. schenckii* encapsulated in an eosinophilic envelope. Gridley fungus stain. × 1440. 704968. (57–2457). **C.** *S. schenckii* in sections of testicular abscess. Gridley fungus stain. × 1440. 321920. (57–2455). **D.** *S. schenckii* in peribronchial nodes of case shown in **C.** Gridley fungus stain. × 1440. (60–1437). **E.** *S. schenckii* in peritoneal exudate of mouse inoculated with recently isolated culture from a lesion of the skin. Observe the similarity of the fungus cells to those shown in the sections from human lesions. Gridley stain. × 1000. 507567. (60-1438). (Emmons, Binford and Utz, Medical Mycology, courtesy of Lea & Febiger)

ulcers which discharge a suppurative brownish red exudate. In a recent report by Londero and associates,[10] a sporotrichotic infection involving a six-year-old female boxer was described in detail and was characterized by multiple nodules (1.4 cm. in diameter and distributed on all parts of the body) with ulcerative centers, raised borders and covered with crust. In another case involving a two-year-old male boxer, lesions were restricted to the head, flank and hind quarters. They had a verrucous appearance and were strikingly similar to the lesions of ringworm.

Infections of other animal species are too uncommon to report in detail or with accuracy. It is of interest that arthritic sporotrichosis has been reported in a boar that was unable to stand on its hind legs;[1] a possible case in the bovine species has been reported by Humphreys and Helmer[7] in which pulmonary lesions were the outstanding findings.

In all cases in which pathologic studies have been undertaken, the primary lesion of sporotrichosis is a granuloma. In veterinary pathology texts,[15,16] the microscopic findings are reported to be: a granulomatous inflammatory reaction with a purulent center, surrounded by epithelioid granulation tissue (containing an abundance of epithelioid cells, a few giant cells and lymphocytes), encapsulated by a dense connective tissue capsule. In a comprehensive review of the histopathologic findings of sporotrichosis in man, Lurie[17] reports that the following pathologic reactions are almost constant features of the disease: pseudoepitheliomatous hyperplasia, intraepidermal microabscesses, infiltration by lymphocytes and plasma cells, intradermal microabscesses and perivascular round cell infiltrate at periphery of the lesion. To a lesser degree the following are found in the histopathologic reaction: eosinophils, free giant cells, sporotrichotic granulomata, tuberculoid granulomata, foreign body granulomata, fibrosis and asteroid bodies. The latter structure represents fungal elements in the reaction and consists of a central spore which is usually spherical. Occasionally one may find a single bud and rarely there may be a cluster or chain of three or four spores. When stained by the periodic acid-Schiff method the wall appears to have a double contour. Surrounding the spore there is a variable amount of homogeneous eosinophilic material which has a stellate shape due to angular projections of varying length.

It is worth emphasizing that the demonstration of the organism in biopsy material usually is difficult and unrewarding. The use of specific fungal stains, as periodic acid-Schiff or methenamine-silver, is more helpful in attempts to demonstrate the organism than is the usual hematoxylin and eosin stain. In the tissues, the organism is pleomorphic. It may be oval, rounded or cigar-shaped (Fig. 2–2).

LABORATORY DIAGNOSIS

Direct Microscopic Examination

Direct microscopic examination of exudative material from lesions (and even microscopic examination of biopsy material) usually is unrewarding because of the paucity of organisms present in the purulent exudate or tissue.[3,18] However, attempts should be made; if present, the organisms may be clearly demonstrated with PAS or silver-methenamine stains. Another diagnostic procedure, which employs fluorescein labeled immune globulins, has been reported by Kaplan and Ivens[19] as a simple, rapid and specific method for demonstrating the organism in exudates or tissues.

Culture

This method is a reliable diagnostic procedure for the identification of *S. schenckii*. Exudative material to be cultured should be aspirated from an unopened lesion, employing the usual aseptic techniques, and placed on Sabouraud's agar and Francis' glucose cystine blood agar or brain-heart infusion glucose blood agar. Chloramphenicol and cycloheximide may be incorporated in the culture medium.

S. schenckii is dimorphic. It appears as a budding yeast in the host's tissues and on enriched culture media when grown at 37° C. It grows in a mycelial form when cultured at room temperature. Sabouraud's agar adequately supports mycelia growth, and it is a useful isolation medium.

Mycelial colonies are at first moist (three to seven days) and have a wrinkled or folded surface. A white to greyish aerial mycelium then appears (initially at periphery), and with age becomes yellow and eventually black. There is considerable variation in colony color. Old cultures and those frequently transferred often partially or completely lose their ability to produce pigment.

Microscopically, the mycelium is composed of fine (2 μ in diameter) branching septate hyphae. Delicate, tapered conidiophores rise at right angles from the hyphae (Fig. 2–3). Initially conidia are borne at the tip of the conidiophore in a manner which resembles "flower-like petals." Each conidium is borne on a very delicate sterigma. As sporulation progresses, spores are formed along the sides of the conidiophores and eventually along the hyphae. Conidia are pyriform to oval or nearly spherical and measure 2 to 3 $\times$ 3 to 6 μ.

The tissue or yeast form of *S. schenckii* grows adequately on Francis' glucose cystine agar or blood enriched BHI agar when incubated at 37° C. Colonies appear in a few days. They are yeast-like with a pasty consistency, and with color variations from creamy white to grey to yellowish.

Microscopic examination reveals small round or oval budding cells. Some cells are elongated and have been described as cigar-shaped and have been termed "cigar bodies." The cells are positively stained by Gram's method.

Because there are several nonpathogenic *Sporotrichum species* which resemble *S. schenckii*, it is essential that the tissue form be demonstrated to identify the pathogenic fungus. The mycelial form can be converted to the tissue form by inoculation onto enriched medium and incubation at 37° C. The medium surface must be kept moist. Several transfers may be required to obtain complete conversion. Also, if 0.2 ml. of a dense mycelial suspension is injected intratesticularly into mice, a purulent orchitis results. Pus containing the converted yeast form of the fungus may be expressed from the testes two to three weeks post-injection. Gram-stained smears will show the round yeastlike cells and "cigar bodies."

Pathogenicity Tests

Purulent material obtained aseptically from unopened lesions may be inoculated into experimental animals in the diagnostic regimen for sporotrichosis. Rats, hamsters or mice may be employed for this purpose. The intraperitoneal inoculation of pus or suspensions of cells from cultures into mice causes a peritonitis.[18] In male mice an orchitis may occur within 10 days. The disease in mice tends to be progressive, and disseminated lesions, particularly involving the bones, are characteristic.[3] Microscopic examination of material obtained from infected sites reveals numerous cigar-shaped, gram-positive organisms.

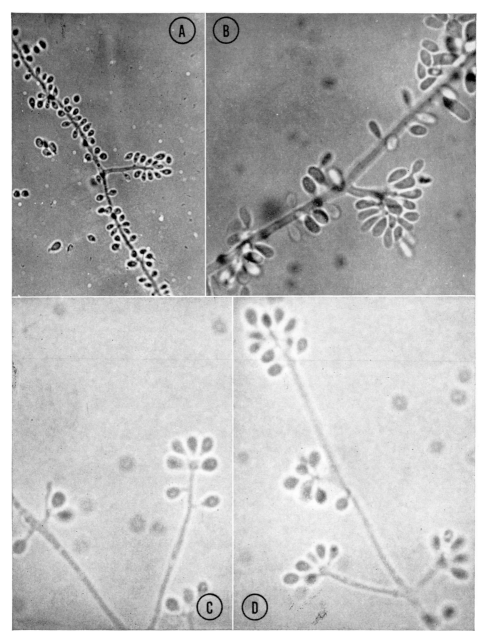

Fig. 2–3. *Sporotrichum schenckii* in culture. **A.** × 400. **B-D.** × 1575. (Emmons, Binford and Utz, Medical Mycology, courtesy of Lea & Febiger)

Immunology

Experimental infection of laboratory animals evokes a weak antibody response which suggests that the slow progression of the disease and its tendency to stay subcutaneous relates more to the low virulence of the organism rather than the host's immunologic ability to localize the infection.[20] In man and experimental animals, antibodies of the complement-fixing, agglutinating and precipitating types have been demonstrated. There is little information regarding the antibody response in domestic animals. The precipitin test appears to be the most sensitive of serologic methods, but it should be noted that cross reactions with other fungi and bacteria may occur. In man, agglutination titers of 1 to 50 are suggestive of an active infection. Reports dealing with an intradermal skin test which employs a heat-killed vaccine or a polysaccharide fraction obtained from the fungus are not available in the veterinary literature. However, in man a delayed (24- to 48-hour, tuberculin-type) reaction may be induced as early as the fifth day following an infection.[18]

DIFFERENTIAL DIAGNOSIS

The presence of subcutaneous nodules or a nodular lymphangitis which ulcerates and drains a thick purulent material is highly suggestive of sporotrichosis. The disease must be differentiated from epizootic lymphangitis (caused by *Histoplasma farciminosum*) which it clinically resembles. In both diseases lesions are similar and develop along the lymphatics of the extremities; however, in epizootic lymphangitis the lesions tend to occur on the mucous membranes of the nostrils and upper respiratory tract. A definitive diagnosis is based on the identification of the organism.

EPIDEMIOLOGY

S. schenckii is a saprophyte in nature and has been isolated from soil, humus plants, fertilizer, sphagnum moss, water and the mouth of normal rat and man as well as from his gastrointestinal tract and tracheobronchial tree.[20] Ahearn and Kaplan[21] recently reported on the isolation of *S. schenckii* from cold-stored frankfurters.

In most cases, a wound infection is the route of entrance of the organism into the host. This situation explains in part the predominance of lesions on the extremities of animals, as the legs are particularly prone to traumatic insults. Bite wounds by rodents, particularly rats, may result in an active infection; finally, it has been suggested that in rare cases the entry of the organism into the body may be by ingestion or inhalation.

The effect of environmental temperature on the disease may be of significant importance. Though hot and humid weather favors the growth of the organism in nature, Mackinnon and Conti-Díaz[22] reported on the inhibitory effect of high ambient temperature on the course of the infection. Young male rats kept at low ambient temperatures, 5 to 20° C., developed lesions in their bones of the paws and tails whereas no lesions developed at these sites when animals were kept at temperatures of 31° C. In addition, a human patient with localized sporotrichosis was cured after treatment with hot dressings.

Sporotrichosis is not a contagious disease and animal-to-man, man-to-man, or man-to-animal transmission should not be anticipated.

TREATMENT

Sporotrichosis is fortunately one of the mycotic infections which may be treated successfully with a number of agents: inorganic iodides, amphotericin B and 2-hydroxystilbamidine. Reports dealing with the beneficial effects of griseofulvin in the treatment of the disease are conflicting: one equine and a number of human cases have been treated successfully with griseofulvin,[8,20] even though the organism is not sensitive to the antibiotic in vitro. Tsubura and Schwarz[23] were not able to demonstrate a beneficial action of the drug when it was administered to experimentally infected mice. Therapeutic failures with griseofulvin have also been reported in man.[20]

The administration of inorganic iodides is a time-honored approach and clinical cures are the rule rather than the exception. How the inorganic iodides bring about their beneficial effect is enigmatic as the organism is capable of multiplying in vitro in a 10-per cent solution of potassium iodide. The known proteolytic activity of inorganic iodides has been suggested as the mechanism by which the drug helps to resolve the infection.[20]

In domestic animals, sodium or potassium iodide often is administered at a dose rate which induces iodinism; at which time the drug is withdrawn for a few days and then administered at lower dose levels. For example, Davis and Worthington[8] gave a nine-year-old thoroughbred stallion a daily dose of 10 gm. potassium iodide per os and 6 gm. sodium iodide intravenously. Within five days iodine intoxication occurred and the dose was dropped to a daily administration of 10 gm. potassium iodide per os. Fishburn and Kelley[9] employed the following regimen in treating a thoroughbred gelding: 2 ounces sodium iodide intravenously (initially) and then repeated in 48 hours, followed by the daily administration of one ounce organic iodide (not specified by the authors) per os for five months. Londero and colleagues[10] treated a six-year-old female boxer by the daily administration 0.5 Gm. potassium iodide (added to the patient's milk) for six weeks, and a two-year-old male boxer by the b.i.d. administration of 25 drops of a saturated solution of potassium iodide per os (before meals) for six weeks. It is worth noting that the results obtained in treating the subcutaneous-lymphatic form of the disease with inorganic iodides are better than those achieved in treating the disseminated form of sporotrichosis. Also, treatment of the disease with iodides is prolonged (weeks to months) and should be continued for four weeks following apparent cure.

Amphotericin B has not been employed in the treatment of domestic animals, though the antibiotic has been shown to inhibit the yeast phase of *S. schenckii* in vitro and has been employed successfully in the treatment of both subcutaneous and disseminated forms of the disease in man.[20] It is possible that intralesional injection of the drug also would be of value in treating localized cutaneous eruptions.

Surgical incision, excision, cauterization, etc. of integumentary lesions are contraindicated as any one of these approaches is often followed by increased suppuration and ulceration.[18]

The topical application of moist hot dressings to cutaneous lesions has been reported to be beneficial in the treatment of sporotrichosis.[22] Forty-minute applications of hot wet towels, t.i.d., to the affected hand and forearm of a human patient for three months resulted in clinical cure.

In summary, (1) inorganic iodides are the drug of choice for the treatment of subcutaneous-lymphatic form of the disease; (2) topical applications of moist hot dressings should be a supplemental therapeutic program in the non-disseminated form of the disease; and (3) inorganic iodides should be tried in the treatment of the disseminated form of sporotrichosis and, if unsuccessful, amphotericin B should be administered intravenously. Therapeutic trials with griseofulvin and the intralesional injection of amphotericin B are worthy of consideration. The proclivity of the organism to remain localized, the slow progression of the disease and the usual success obtained in treatment allow for a good prognosis.

REFERENCES

1. Smith, H. C.: Arthritic Sporotrichosis in a Boar. V.M./S.A.C., *60* (1965): 164–165.
2. Saliba, A. M., Matera, E. A., and Moreno, G.: Sporotrichosis in a Chimpanzee. Mod. Vet. Practice, *49* (1968): 74.
3. Emmons, C. W., Binford, C. H., and Utz, J. P.: *Medical Mycology*. 2nd edition, Philadelphia, Lea & Febiger, 1970.
4. Ainsworth, G. C. and Austwick, P. K. C.: *Fungal Diseases of Animals*. Farnham Royal, Bucks, England, Commonwealth Agricultural Bureaux, 1959.
5. Curasson, G.: *Traité de Pathologie Exotique Vétérnaire et Comparée*. Vol. 2., Maladies Microbiennes, 2nd edition, Paris, Vigot Frères, 1942.
6. Saunders, L. Z.: Systemic Fungus Infections in Animals: A Review. Cornell Vet., *38* (1948): 213–238.
7. Humphreys, F. A. and Helmer, D. E.: Pulmonary Sporotrichosis in a Cattle Beast. Canad. J. Comp. Med., *7* (1943): 199–204.
8. Davis, H. H. and Worthington, W. E.: Equine Sporotrichosis. J. Amer. Vet. Med. Ass., *145* (1964): 692–693.
9. Fishburn, F. and Kelley, D. C.: Sporotrichosis in a Horse. J. Amer. Vet. Med. Ass., *151* (1967): 45–46.
10. Londero, A. T., de Castro, R. M., and Fischman, O.: Two Cases of Sporotrichosis in Dogs in Brazil. Sabouraudia, *3* (1964): 273–275.
11. Hull, T. G.: *Diseases Transmitted from Animals to Man*. 4th edition, Springfield, Charles C Thomas, Publisher, 1955.
12. Ditchfield, J.: *Equine Medicine and Surgery*. 1st edition. Wheaton, American Veterinary Publ., Inc., 1963.
13. Blood, D. C. and Henderson, J. A.: *Veterinary Medicine*. 3rd edition, Baltimore, Williams & Wilkins Company, 1968.
14. Král, F. and Schwartzman, R. M.: *Veterinary and Comparative Dermatology*. 2nd edition, Philadelphia, J. B. Lippincott Company, 1964.
15. Smith, H. A., Jones, T. C., and Hunt, R. D.: *Veterinary Pathology*. 4th edition, Philadelphia, Lea & Febiger, 1972.
16. Jubb, K. V. F. and Kennedy, P. C.: *Pathology of Domestic Animals*. Vol. 1, 2nd edition, New York and London, Academic Press Inc., 1970.
17. Lurie, H. I.: Histopathology of Sporotrichosis. Arch. Path., *75* (1963): 421–437.
18. Conant, N. F., Smith, D. T., Baker, R. D., Callaway, J. L., and Martin, D. S.: *Manual of Clinical Mycology*. 2nd edition, Philadelphia and London, W. B. Saunders Company, 1954.
19. Kaplan, W. and Ivens, M. S.: Fluorescent Antibody Staining of Sporotrichum Schenckii in Cultures and Clinical Material. J. Invest. Derm., *35* (1960): 151–159.
20. Hildick-Smith, G., Blank, H., and Sarkany, I.: *Fungus Diseases and Their Treatment*. Boston, Little, Brown & Co., 1964.
21. Ahearn, D. G. and Kaplan, W.: Occurrence of Sporotrichum Schenckii on a Cold-Stored Meat Product. Amer. J. Epidemiology, *89* (1969): 116–124.
22. Mackinnon, J. E. and Conti-Díaz, I. A.: The Effect of Temperature on Sporotrichosis. Sabouraudia, *2* (1962): 56–59.
23. Tsubura, E. and Schwarz, J.: Treatment of Experimental Sporotrichosis in Mice with Griseofulvin and Amphotericin B. Antibiot. Chemother. (N.Y.), *10* (1960): 753–757.

CHAPTER 3 | Rhinosporidiosis

Rhinosporidiosis is a chronic infection of the mucous membranes of the nasal cavity, characterized by polypoid growths and caused by *Rhinosporidium seeberi*. The disease has been reported in cattle, horses, mules,[1,2] dogs,[3,4] goats,[5] and geese and ducks.[6]

HISTORY, GEOGRAPHIC DISTRIBUTION AND PREVALENCE

The initial reports of rhinosporidiosis appeared in the literature at the end of the nineteenth century and dealt with the disease in man. Seeber described the causative agent in 1900, and the first animal case was reported in the horse by Zschokke in 1913,[7] in cattle by Vogelsang in 1923[8] and later by Ayyar[9] and Rao,[10] and in mules by Quinlan and DeKoch[11] in 1926. It was not until 1923 that *R. seeberi* was identified by Ashworth[12] as a fungus. In the more recent literature, a number of reports have come from South America[4,13,14,15] and from the United States.[16,17,18]

The disease is widely distributed throughout the world. It is endemic in Argentina, Ceylon and India. Sporadic cases have been reported from Australia, Brazil, South Africa and the United States.

No figures regarding the incidence of the disease are available, but it is generally considered to be a rare infection of domestic animals in the United States. In both man and animals a prevalence of the disease in males has been reported.[19,10] In man, there is an age predilection of the disease for children and young adults. This has not been reported in animals. The parallel incidence of the disease in animals and man varies with locality: in South India, the disease in both species parallels one another; in humid climates of India, human cases are frequent but animal cases are rare; in dry areas of India, a few cases have been reported in man but none in animals; and in the central provinces of India, no cases have been reported in animals but human cases are frequent. In general, the disease in man is more severe than in animals and disseminated lesions have been reported in man only.[5]

CLINICAL SIGNS AND PATHOLOGY

The primary lesion of rhinosporidiosis is a polyp, which may be pedunculated or sessile, pink in color and usually no larger than 3 cm. in diameter. The growth is

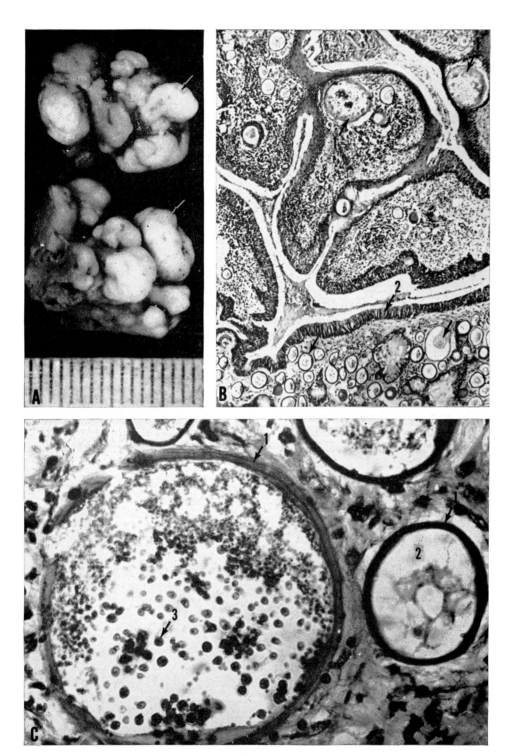

Fig. 3–1. Rhinosporidiosis. **A.** Polypoid masses from nasal mucosa of a horse. **B.** Section ($\times$ 100) of one of the polyps. *Rhinosporidium seeberi* containing endospore (**1**) or as empty cysts, elevating the mucous membrane (**2**). **C.** The organism ($\times$ 600); note thick wall (**1**), empty organisms (**2**), and others containing small and large (**3**) endospores. AFIP 233008. Contributor: Col. M. W. Hale. (Smith, Jones and Hunt, Veterinary Pathology, courtesy of Lea & Febiger)

often soft and friable, bleeds easily, and has a lobulated surface which creates a cauliflowerlike appearance. Small white specks (sporangia) may be seen on its surface. Most reports of the disease in domestic animals have described the polypoid growths as occurring in the nasal cavity (Fig. 3–1A); but some authors[1] have indicated that the conjunctival sac, vagina and various parts of the integumentary system (particularly the ears) may be involved. The growths may be singular or multiple but generally involve only one nasal cavity. If sufficiently large to block the nasal cavity, the initial manifestations of the disease may be stertorous breathing (inspiratory) or severe dyspnea. A blood-stained, mucopurulent nasal discharge also may be an early presenting sign of the disease.[20] The general health of the animal usually is not affected by the presence of the polyps in the nasal cavity and internal dissemination of the infection has not been reported in animals.

Microscopic examination (Fig. 3–1B, C) of the polyps reveals a papillomatous epithelium (Figs. 3–2, 3–3) which is usually intact; it may be hyperplastic and contain sporangia.[18] The bulk of the polyp consists of a stroma of fibrous or fibromyxoid tissue.[3] Numerous sporangia or spores are imbedded in this fibrillar or fibromyxomatous tissue.[2,16] An increased vascularity may be evident also. The cellular infiltrate is quite variable in extent and type. The principal inflammatory cells are lymphocytes and epithelioid cells. It generally is agreed that the evacuation of the sporangia excites an intense cellular reaction; neutrophils, eosinophils, red blood cells, giant cells, histiocytes and mast cells may be observed when the wall of the sporangium is fragmented.[2,3,16,21] *Rhinosporidium seeberi* usually is seen readily in tissues stained with hematoxylin and eosin. The walls of maturing sporangia and the spores also are stained positively by Gridley's fungus stain and the periodic acid-Schiff reaction. (A description of the organism as it appears in tissue sections follows.)

LABORATORY DIAGNOSIS

Direct Microscopic Examination

R. seeberi has not been grown in culture* nor have laboratory animals been infected experimentally. Thus, the only method of diagnosing the disease is by the demonstration of the spores or sporangia in the nasal exudate or in the tissues. Spores (7 μ in diameter) and sporangia (300 to 400 μ in diameter) may be squeezed with a forceps from biopsy material with gentle pressure into a drop of water and visualized microscopically.[19]

In the tissues, an infecting spore appears as a round body (7 μ in diameter) with a chitinous wall, a nucleus and a karyosome.[2,19] The spore enlarges to a diameter of 100 μ at which time a cellulose layer is deposited within the chitinous wall. Numerous nuclear divisions account for this growth and the fungal structure at this stage is referred to as a sporangium. As maturation continues, the sporangium grows to a diameter of 300 to 350 μ and contains 16,000 to 20,000 spores within its walls. At a single point, the wall of the sporangium thins to form a pore from which the spores eventually escape. The size of the spores within a sporangium is quite variable. Mature spores (7 μ in diameter) appear to accumulate near the pore while smaller ones (5 μ or less) may be seen on the opposite side of the sporangium.

* *R. seeberi* has not been grown in a mycelial form. However, Grover[22] obtained maturation of spores and sporangia in biopsy material placed in synthetic liquid medium T.C.199.

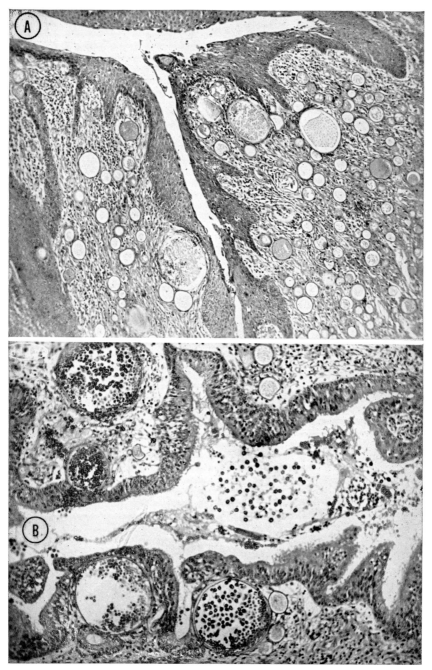

Fig. 3–2. Rhinosporidiosis. **A.** Section through the surface of a nasal polypoid lesion. Observe the epithelial hyperplasia and the numerous cysts in the chronically inflamed stroma. H & E. × 90. 750521. (57–13229). **B.** Section showing a cleft in a nasal polypoid lesion. The pseudostratified epithelium is inflamed. The proximity of the maturing sporangia to the surface is demonstrated. Rupture of a sporangium through the epidermis was probably responsible for the spores which are present in the mucoid exudate in the cleft space. H & E. × 120. (62093). (Emmons, Binford and Utz, Medical Mycology, courtesy of Lea & Febiger)

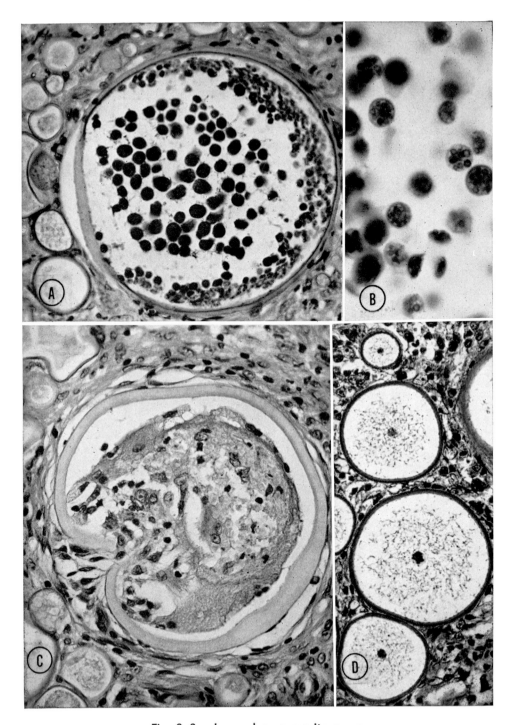

Fig. 3–3.   Legend on opposite page.

Culture

All attempts to grow *R. seeberi* on culture media have been unsuccessful.*

Pathogenicity Tests

No laboratory animal has been infected experimentally.

Immunology

Little is known regarding the immunologic aspects of rhinosporidiosis.

DIFFERENTIAL DIAGNOSIS

Stertorous breathing or a mucopurulent nasal discharge (unilateral) should direct the clinician to an examination of the nasal cavity. The appearance of polyps (singular or multiple, no greater than 3 cm. in diameter, sessile or pedunculated, speckled with minute white spots) is highly suggestive of rhinosporidiosis. A definitive diagnosis depends upon the demonstration of spores or sporangium in the exudate or biopsy specimen. A foreign body in a nasal cavity may produce some of the clinical signs mentioned. Nasal granulomas in cattle caused by other fungi (*Helminthosporium*) or flukes (*Schistosoma*) must be differentiated from rhinosporidiosis on the basis of demonstrating or culturing the respective organisms.

EPIDEMIOLOGY

Rhinosporidiosis, though it affects both man and domestic animals, is not a contagious disease and there is no evidence that animal-to-animal, animal-to-man, or man-to-man transmission occurs. The epidemiology of this disease remains an enigma. The natural habitat of the organism is unknown. It has been suggested that *R. seeberi* is a saprophyte in water or that aquatic animals play a part in the maintenance of the organism in nature. Reddy and Lakshminarayana,[23] in an extensive study of the epidemiology of the disease, were not able to support this hypothesis. Examination of water, fish, snails, cyclops, silt and manure from areas in which the disease was endemic failed to reveal the organism. Fish and snails reared in aquaria, the water of which contained the organism, were not infected. Also, attempts to infect fish and snails artificially with *R. seeberi* failed.

* *R. seeberi* has not been grown in a mycelial form. However, Grover[22] obtained maturation of spores and sporangia in biopsy material placed in synthetic liquid medium T.C.199.

Fig. 3–3.   Rhinosporidiosis.   **A.** A mature sporangium in the stroma of a polypoid lesion. The maturing spores (endospores) are apically and centrally located. The stroma contains many smaller cysts which represent "trophic" stages of the fungus. H & E. $\times$ 400. 750521. (62–904). **B.** Mature spores from a sporangium similar to the one shown in **A.** Observe the small globular bodies within the spores. These bodies are usually reddish pink in the H & E. stain. H & E. $\times$ 920. (57–13763). **C.** Granulomatous reactive tissue now fills the cavity of a cyst from which the spores have been extruded. The reactive cells within the cyst are continuous with the pericystic tissue through a small opening which presumably is the pore through which spores escaped. H & E. $\times$ 300. (62–905). **D.** Developing "trophic" stages of the fungus in a nasal lesion. In this field the trophic stages range from 25 to 100 μ in diameter. The cysts contain nuclei and nutritional material, but no spores. H & E. $\times$ 40. 134695. (62–907). (Emmons, Binford and Utz, Medical Mycology, courtesy of Lea & Febiger)

The suggestion that the disease is an airborne infection (and that the organism is carried by dust to the nasal cavity) has never been supported by evidence. Trauma, however, may play a predisposing role in infections by this fungus: Rao[10] has observed that there is a higher incidence of the disease in male draft oxen whose nasal septa are pierced for a nose string than in animals not subjected to this procedure. In addition, lesions occurring in these oxen usually appear on the margin of the string hole. Also there may be an association between rhinosporidiosis and nasal infections by *Schistosoma nasale*.

Few infectious diseases today have such large gaps of information pertaining to the natural habitat of the organism, mode of infection, cultural characteristics and immunology. Fortunately the disease, though chronic, runs a benign course in domestic animals and its apparent rare occurrence in this country will not allow for intensive investigations necessary to give us a better understanding of it.

TREATMENT

Rhinosporidiosis is best treated by surgical excision of the polyps. This approach for most animal patients has a successful end result though recurrence of the lesion may occur. Griseofulvin is of no value in the treatment of the disease and the reports dealing with the use of amphotericin B are too limited to suggest efficacy.

REFERENCES

1. Král, F. and Schwartzman, R. M.: *Veterinary and Comparative Dermatology.* 2nd edition, Philadelphia, J. B. Lippincott Company, 1964.
2. Ainsworth, G. C. and Austwick, P. K. C.: *Fungal Diseases of Animals.* Farnham Royal, Bucks, England, Commonwealth Agricultural Bureaux, 1959.
3. Jubb, K. V. F. and Kennedy, P. C.: *Pathology of Domestic Animals.* Vol. 1, 2nd edition, New York and London, Academic Press Inc., 1970.
4. Nino, F. L. and Freire, R. S.: Existence of Endemic Focus of Rhinosporidiosis in Chaco Province, Argentina. Mycopath. and Mycol. Appl., *24* (1964): 92–102.
5. Datla, S.: Rhinosporidium Seeberi—Its Cultivation and Identity. Indian J. Vet. Sci. and Anim. Husb., *35* (1965): 1–17.
6. Fain, A. and Herm, V.: Two Cases of Nasal Rhinospordiosis in a Wild Goose and a Wild Duck. Mycopathologia, *8* (1957): 54–61.
7. Zschokke, E.: Em Rhinosporidium beim Pferd. Schweiz. Arch. f. Tierheilk., *55* (1913): 641–650.
8. Vogelsang, E. G.: Conf. Sudamericana. Hyg. Microbiol. Patol., *2* (1923): 305 (Quoted by Saunders, L. Z.: Cornell Vet., *38* (1948): 230).
9. Ayyar, V. F.: Rhinosporidiosis in Equines. Indian J. Vet. Sci. and Anim. Husb., *2* (1932): 49–52.
10. Rao, M. A. N.: Rhinosporidiosis in Bovines in the Madras Presidency, With a Discussion of the Probable Modes of Infection. Indian J. Vet. Sci. and Anim. Husb., *8* (1938): 187–198.
11. Quinlan, J. and De Koch, G.: Report of Two Cases of Rhinosporidiosis in Mules in South Africa. S. Afr. J. Sci., *23* (1926): 589–594.
12. Ashworth, J. H.: Ozi Rhinosporidium Seeberi (Wernicke, 1963) With Special Reference to Its Sporulation and Affinities. Trans. Roy. Soc. Edinburgh, *53* (1922): 301–342 (Pt. 2).
13. Schlögel, F. and Curial, O.: Rhinosporidiosis in Two Horses in Brazil. Arch. Biol. (Curitiba), *11* (1956): 3–7.
14. Laffont, H. E.: Rhinosporidiosis in Four Horses in Argentina. Gac. Vet. (B. Air.) *23* (1961): 379–382.
15. Barros, S. S. and Santiago, C. M.: Sobre o Primeiro Caso de Rhinosporidiose Bovina no Brazil. Rev. Med. Vet (B. Air.), *3* (1968): 225–238.

16. Smith, H. A. and Frankson, M. C.:   Rhinosporidiosis in a Texas Horse.   Southwest. Vet. *15* (1961): 22–24.
17. Smith, H. A. and Frankson, M. C.:   A Second Case of Rhinosporidiosis in a Texas Horse.   Southwest. Vet. *17*, (1963): 17.
18. Myers, D. D., Simon, J. and Case, M. T.:   Rhinosporidiosis in a Horse.   J. Amer. Vet. Med. Ass., *145* (1964): 345–47.
19. Conant, N. F., Smith, D. T., Baker, R. D., Callaway, J. L. and Martin, D. S.:   *Manual of Clinical Mycology.*   2nd edition, Philadelphia and London, W. B. Saunders Co., 1954.
20. Blood D. C. and Henderson, J. A.:   *Veterinary Medicine.*   3rd edition, Baltimore, Williams & Wilkins Company, 1968.
21. Smith, H. A., Jones, T. C. and Hunt, R. D.:   *Veterinary Pathology.*   4th edition, Philadelphia, Lea & Febiger, 1972.
22. Grover, S.:   *Rhinosporidium Seeberi;* A Preliminary Study of the Morphology and Life Cycle. Sabouraudia, *7* (1970–4): 249–251.
23. Reddy, D. G. and Lakshminarayana, C. S.:   Investigation Into Transmission, Growth and Serology in Rhinosporidiosis.   Indian J. Med. Res., *50* (1962): 363–370.

CHAPTER **4** | Phycomycosis and Mycetoma

Phycomycosis

Phycomycosis is a granulomatous disease affecting a variety of animals and man caused by fungi of the class *Phycomycetes*. Members of the family *Mucoraceae* belong in this class, and phycomycosis includes the disease sometimes termed mucormycosis.

HISTORY, GEOGRAPHIC DISTRIBUTION AND PREVALENCE

Theobold Smith first described a malady of horses occurring in Florida during the early 1890s.[1] The disease was known locally as "leeches," because horsemen thought the elongated masses of necrotic tissue within the granulomatous lesions were leeches (*Hirudinea*) which had invaded the tissues while the horses were standing in water. At about the same time, a clinically similar disease of horses called "bursattee" had been recognized in India.[2]

In 1903, de Haan and Hoogkamer[3] described a similar equine disease in Indonesia which they called "hyphomycosis destruens"; a nonsporulating phycomycete isolated from the lesions was named *Hyphomyces destruens*. In Indonesia in 1925, *Basidiobolus ranarum* was isolated from a granulomatous lesion on the leg of a mare;[4] this apparently is the only record of animal infection with this fungus. However, it has been recovered from human cases of phycomycosis in Indonesia and Africa.[5] *Mucor pusillus* was isolated from a nodule in a horse in 1928.[6] This is the only record of a member of the genus *Mucor* being identified in equine phycomycosis.

More recently, a condition resembling and probably identical with "leeches" and "hyphomycosis destruens" has been described in Florida and Texas horses by Bridges and Emmons.[7] They repeatedly isolated *Hyphomyces destruens* from the lesions and described the fungus in detail. These authors, in collaboration with Romane, have described a phycomycosis of horses caused by *Entomophthora coronata* which has a predilection for the nasal mucosa and for the skin adjacent to the oral and nasal mucosa;[8] a complete description of this fungus was recorded in another publication.[9]

48

Bridges[10] discussed the association of the early Florida cases of "leeches" with lakes and muck ponds in which the horses waded during grazing. Similar conditions seem to contribute to the etiology of *H. destruens* phycomycosis in Texas, thus a possible geographic limitation exists. Interestingly, a disease known as "malzo" is markedly like *H. destruens* phycomycosis and afflicts horses in Haiti. It is more prevalent in the Artibonite Valley where it causes serious economic losses. An association with tethering horses along irrigation canal banks and with pasturing in rice stubble has been noted.[11]

Most writers credit Rivolta[12] (1885) with the first report of canine phycomycosis, although the disease was not well-documented until Gleiser[13] described two cases in 1953. Pathologic changes were found largely in the kidney of one and the gastric fundus in the other. Only three other canine cases were reported prior to 1970.[14,15,16] A world literature review would indicate that canine phycomycosis is very rare, but it is noteworthy that three cases were recently diagnosed at Texas A. & M. University by Heller and colleagues[17] within a 60-day time span. Also, Bridges has records of 11 other unreported cases of canine phycomycosis in the TAMU Department of Pathology files.

Obviously the disease is more prevalent than is generally recognized and a need exists for documentation of these cases. More importantly, precise cultural identification of the causal fungi—all too often lacking in reports of animal mycotic diseases—is needed to help clarify the etiology.

A multitude of cases of bovine phycomycotic diseases has been reported. In

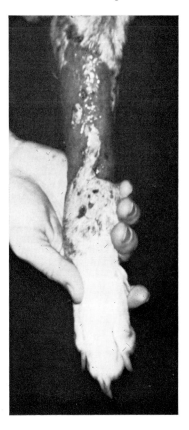

Fig. 4–1. Phycomycosis (mucormycosis) of limb of dog from which *Mucor pusillus* was repeatedly isolated.

1935, Jungherr[18] incriminated fungi of the genera *Aspergillus, Rhizopus* and *Mucor* in abortions and other reproductive problems. Gleiser's report in 1953[13] of caseocalcareous lesions in bronchial and mediastinal lymph nodes included a comprehensive literature review to that date. His case was included in the study by Davis and associates[19] of 12 additional bovine cases. The problem of grossly differentiating mycotic lesions from those of tuberculosis and other granulomas was presented.

Mucoraceous hyphae, found in severe abomasal ulcers of young calves, have been described by Gitter and Austwick.[20] Fungal isolation attempts were unsuccessful. Mycotic abomasitis was an observation of Cordes and Shortridge also.[21] These workers reported finding fungal hyphae in tissue sections of 116 cases of bovine systemic mycosis. Mycotic lesions were described in a great variety of organs, most commonly in mycotic placentitis and/or acute mycotic pneumonia. Cordes and Shortridge stated that mixed infections occurred in these diseases and that cultural isolates may not be representative of fungi in lesions.

These points are recorded here only to point out and emphasize the need for studies to clarify the etiologic role of these fungi. As was previously stated, precise cultural identifications must be made. Predisposing factors, possibly multiple, are no doubt involved, and these should be considered and recorded in all reports of phycomycotic disease of animals.

These criteria were met in a recent report of rhino-orbital phycomycosis in a monkey (*Macaca mulatta*) with suspected predisposing diabetes.[22] Uncontrolled diabetes, bone marrow hypoplasia, malignancies and prolonged treatment with antibiotics or corticosteroids are considered to be important predisposing causes of this disease in man.[5,22,23] Gastric infarction in a rhesus monkey resulting from mycotic infection was thought to be associated with an extensive period of treatment with orally administered antibiotics.[23]

Spontaneous pulmonary disease caused by *Mucor pusillus* has been reported in a harp seal.[24] Interestingly, the isolate produced experimental pneumonia in rabbits made diabetic with intravenous administration of alloxan.

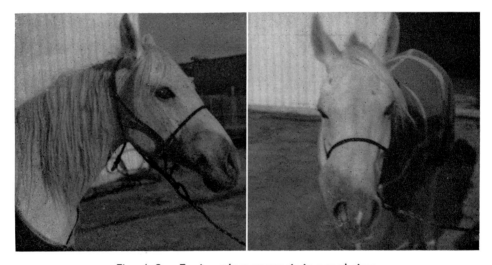

Fig. 4–2.   Equine phycomycosis in nasal sinus.

Because of the wide distribution of the phycomycetes in nature, there apparently are no geographic limitations to the diseases they may cause in man and animals. Because these fungi occur commonly as laboratory contaminants, many laboratorians are reluctant to report them as possible pathogens. Thus, the true prevalence of animal phycomycosis is obscure.

CLINICAL SIGNS AND PATHOLOGY

Adequate clinical descriptions of animal phycomycosis have been recorded only for the horse. In other animal species, the diagnosis has been made most often at necropsy where the lesions were found in a variety of organs. Sometimes the lesions could be related retrospectively to clinical illness although commonly such associations have been vague.

Equine phycomycosis is usually seen as an area or areas of exuberant granulation (most often on the limbs between the hoof and knee or hock) but may be found on the ventral abdomen, neck, lips and skin surrounding the nostrils. Most develop rather slowly at loci thought to have been previously traumatized, often following wire cuts. Occasionally extension of the granulation is quite rapid, especially on the legs, and lameness results when functional structures become involved. Purulent exudates may drain from openings on the surface of the lesion.

The animal may traumatize or destroy part of the lesion by biting or licking, apparently as a result of severe pruritus. Lesions of the nostril may cause inspiratory dyspnea; those on the lips may impair prehension.

Bridges has described comprehensively the gross and microscopic pathology of the lesions:

> The superficial surface of the granulation tissue frequently is hemorrhagic due to trauma inflicted by the horse. Although the ulcerated tissue occasionally may extend some distance above the edge of the skin, it usually remains reasonably flush with it. There is sufficient peripheral subcutaneous extension of the lesion to raise the skin which, along with trauma of the new tissue by the horse, keeps them at similar levels. In more advanced lesions, small sinuses drain pus from the deeper foci of infection and hard, yellow irregular masses of necrotic tissue may be expressed from them. These frequently are found on a medicated bandage when it is removed. Occasionally, one of these pieces of necrotic tissue may be found anchored firmly in the tissue but protruding slightly on the ulcerated surface.
>
> Incision of the lesions reveals firm, fibrous tissue with cross sections of the sinuses and necrotic masses which vary from less than one-half mm. to several mm. in diameter and up to six cm. long. These smaller ones are difficult to see with the unaided eye. The pieces of necrotic tissue from the more fulminant lesions frequently branch and rebranch in a form suggestive of blood vessels. The tendons and bones ordinarily are not invaded, but the tendon sheaths may be.
>
> Histologically, in the more advanced lesions there is granulation tissue of varying maturity surrounding a sinus in which a cross section of the necrotic tissue is embedded in purulent exudate containing numerous macrophages and occasional giant cells. Eosinophils are extremely numerous, especially in the superficial parts of the lesions, and in and about the sinuses. Fungi are found within the necrotic tissue.
>
> Studies of the early foci of necrosis reveal that they begin as areas of coagulative necrosis surrounding the hyphae. Necrotic eosinophils also are numerous. Many of the larger masses, when examined at the proper time, will be found to contain blood vessels in their centers, thus explaining the branching patterns seen. The fungus can be seen as branching, occasionally septate hyphae which are scattered throughout the larger foci of necrosis and in the centers of the smaller ones. The hyphae frequently are numerous in the necrotic blood vessels.[10]

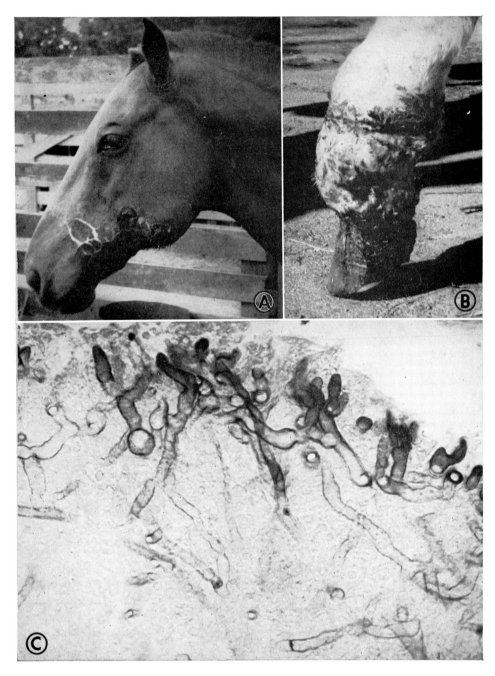

Fig. 4–3. Hyphomycosis destruens. **A, B.** Clinical aspects. **C.** *Hyphomyces destruens* in abscess. $\times$ 700. (Bridges and Emmons, A phycomycosis of horses caused by *Entomophthora coronata*, courtesy of the Journal of the American Veterinary Medical Association)

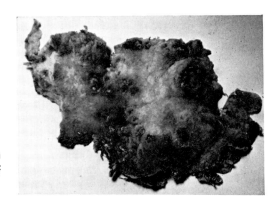

Fig. 4–4. Mass of granulation tissue removed from forelimb of horse with phycomycosis.

LABORATORY DIAGNOSIS

The phycomycetes are common in nature and are encountered often as laboratory contaminants. Many mycologists have stated that these organisms may be secondary invaders and that they are very rarely primary pathogens. Conant[25] advocated that diagnosis of phycomycotic disease be made "reluctantly and only when the evidence is overwhelming." Dodge[26] had previously expressed a similar view.

Gleiser confirmed the pathogenic potential of these fungi in animals, and he stated:

> The fungus was incorporated in a marked granulomatous reaction and was actually being phagocytized by multinucleated giant cells. In none of these cases, even in specially stained sections, was there evidence of another etiological agent which could have been responsible for the severe reactive changes. It is difficult to conceive of a contaminant so intimately associated with the violent pathological process described.

The laboratory has the responsibility of culturing and identifying a potential fungal pathogen. When this supports the histopathologic demonstration of tissue invasion, the diagnosis is secure.

Direct Microscopic Examination

Scrapings from mucosal surfaces and granulomatous lesions should be examined for the presence of broad, aseptate mycelium.

Culture

Sabouraud dextrose agar is a satisfactory isolation medium. It restricts most bacterial contaminants and this feature may be enhanced by the addition of antibacterial antibiotics. Cycloheximide must not be incorporated in the medium; the phycomycetes are sensitive to this antibiotic.

Species identification of the phycomycetes is difficult. They should be referred to a mycologist with an interest or specialty in this fungal group. However, identification of the genera is not difficult and interested students soon develop a remarkable efficiency. Ajello and his associates have published an excellent identification guide which is readily available.[5]

Pathogenicity Tests

Experimental infections of animals are not useful in laboratory diagnosis.

Immunology

Little is known regarding the host's ability to defend against phycomycotic disease. These fungi are generally considered to be apathogenic, yet under certain conditions they are capable of becoming established in tissue, causing severe pathologic changes and occasionally fatal disease. Predisposing factors which alter the normal physiologic status appear to be quite important. Some workers believe that in phycomycosis and some other mycotic diseases, an immunologic defect is necessary for the establishment of an infection.

DIFFERENTIAL DIAGNOSIS

Early and slowly progressing lesions of equine phycomycosis may have minute foci of necrosis with little purulent exudate and may be confused with invasive squamous cell carcinoma or cutaneous habronemiasis. In cutaneous habronemiasis, the yellow foci of necrosis and inflammation seldom are larger than a grain of rice, and they tend to regress spontaneously in the absence of repeated infection which usually stops during the colder weather.[10]

A recent observation[27] that microfilaria (*Onchocerca cervicalis*) can very often be demonstrated in skin biopsy sections of horses with skin lesions suggestive of mycotic infection is worthy of consideration. It appears significant that the parasites are not occasionally present or in low numbers; if the fresh biopsy specimen is placed in saline for a time, organisms by the hundreds migrate from it. They have not been found in normal skin, and a possible co-etiologic role is an interesting speculation. Equine microfilarial pityriasis has been attributed to *O. cervicalis*.[28]

EPIDEMIOLOGY

The phycomycetes are widely disseminated in nature, and man and animals are more or less constantly exposed to them. They are found in soil, water, food and decomposing organic matter where they exist in a free-living state.[24]

The predisposing factors which render animals susceptible to phycomycotic disease need extensive study and documentation. The disease is not transmitted from individual to individual or from animals to man.

Mycetoma

The term mycetoma is generally applied to those tumefactions, usually of the extremities, which are caused by fungi of the classes *Ascomycetes* and *Deuteromycetes* (eumycotic mycetomas). The tumors are quite chronic, most often involve

---

Fig. 4–5. Nasal granuloma of cattle. **A.** Polypoid masses on nasal septum. (Davis, Nasal Swelling in a Bovine, courtesy of the Journal of the American Veterinary Medical Association). **B.** Section of a nasal granuloma, H & E. × 400. Note fungal organisms (**1**) and eosinophils (**2**). (Smith, Jones and Hunt, Veterinary Pathology, courtesy of Lea & Febiger)

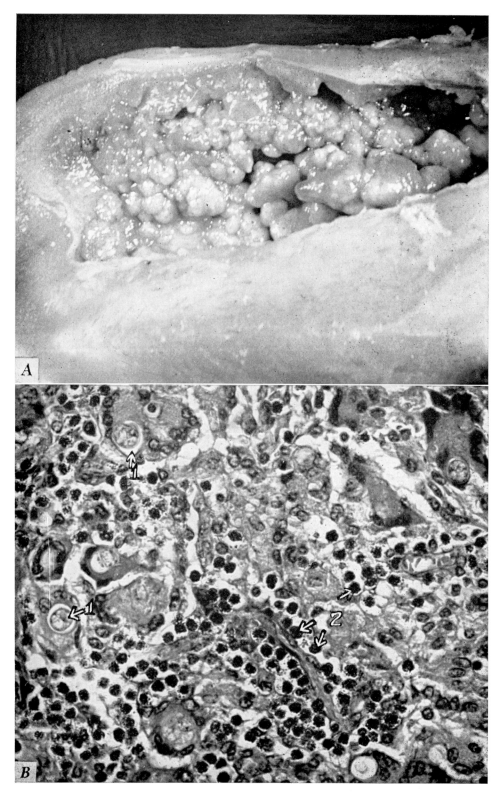

Fig. 4–5. Legend on opposite page.

skin, subcutaneous tissue, fascia and bone, and they contain abscesses and multiple draining sinuses. The exudate and lesions contain granules (colonies of fungal hyphae with or without spores) which vary in size, color and texture with the various etiologic agents.*

Actinomycotic mycetomas, caused by fungi of the family *Actinomycetaceae*, are similar clinically. These are discussed in Chapters 11 and 12.

Historically, mycetoma in man was first reported from India, and most of the early cases were found in the province of Madura. The disease became known as "Madura foot" and "maduromycosis." Both names imply a geographic limitation which is invalid. In man, mycetoma is widely distributed geographically, however, most cases occur in tropical and subtropical areas of the Americas, northern Africa and southern Asia.

All known animal cases of eumycotic mycetoma, with one exception, have occurred in the United States. In contrast, relatively few human cases have been reported in North America. Several other differences in the disease of man and animals are of interest.

A great variety of fungi have been incriminated as etiologic agents of mycetoma in man.[29] Few animal cases have had the causative agent identified, however *Curvularia geniculata* and *Helminthosporium speciferum* have been identified as causing mycetomas in several animal species.[30] Both of these fungi are basically saprophytes and are common in the environment of animals and man, yet they have not been incriminated in human mycetomas.

In the United States, the most frequent etiologic agent of human eumycotic mycetoma is *Allescheria boydii*, an ascomycete that has been isolated from both soil and sewage.[31] This hyaline fungus forms light-colored granules in pus; the majority of animal mycetomas have produced dark-colored granules.[32] Recently two cases of *A. boydii* in dogs, both with abdominal involvement, were reported.[31,32]

These recent reports may indicate that the many other genera and species of fungi that cause mycetoma in man may have a similar capability in animals also. The almost complete lack of reports of animal mycetomas from areas of the world where the disease is most often diagnosed in man probably reflects both the economic importance of animals and lack of interest by mycologists and veterinarians in those areas. Only the three fungus species which have been identified in animal mycetomas will be described.

Allescheria boydii

Allescheria boydii is rapid-growing and initially produces a white, cottony aerial mycelium. With age (two or more weeks), the aerial mycelium becomes brownish grey. Reverse pigment is grey black.

Microscopically, a moderately broad, septate mycelium is observed. Unicellular, oval- to pear-shaped conidia (6 by 9 μ) are attached to their conidiophores by broad, flat bases. Occasionally the conidiophores occur in bundles (coremia).

Some isolates produce sexual, fruiting bodies called perithecia or cleistothecia which represent the perfect stage of *A. boydii*. They may be formed on the agar

---

* Both usage and semantics of definitions have established that mycetomas should produce granules. Fungal granulomas of bovine nasal mucous membranes have been reported twice in the United States.[33,34] Because granules were not formed in the granulomas, some workers have excluded these cases in tabulating the known animal cases of mycetoma.[30]

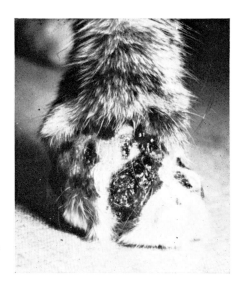

Fig. 4–6.   Granuloma in foot of cat
caused by *Helminthosporium* species.

surface or deep in the agar where they appear as small black specks.   The cleistothecia are dark, thin-walled structures (50–200 μ) which contain delicate asci and
ascospores.   The ascospores are yellowish and oval and are slightly smaller than
the conidia.

Curvularia geniculata

Curvularia geniculata grows rapidly on Sabouraud agar.   The aerial mycelium is
cottony and white in color at first but quickly becomes grey to brown, and finally
black.   The periphery of the colony is thin and lightly pigmented.   Concentric rings
of alternating light brown and black color are produced on reverse.

Microscopically, abundant fusiform, dark brown conidiophores have three to
four septa and a tendency to curve slightly on their long axes.   In Bridges' isolate,
the third cell from the base was larger and darker than the rest and slightly bulged
on one side.   The end cells were almost hyaline.[29]

Helminthosporium spp.

The rapidly growing colony is at first grey in color, then forms a black, depressed
central area with a raised greyish periphery.

Microscopically, the mycelium, conidiophores and conidia are dark brown in
color.[25]   The conidiophore develops as a branch from the mycelium and becomes
swollen on the terminal and may appear knotted or twisted.   The conidia may be
single or multiple and are formed laterally on the swollen end of the conidiophore.
The conidia have a remarkable resemblance to segmented helminth eggs.

TREATMENT

For both phycomycosis and mycetoma radical surgical intervention appears to
offer the best or optimum chance for clinical cure.   Surgery should be performed
early in the course of the disease before structures are invaded.   It is not unusual
for lesions to recur after excision.

Some equine practitioners use so-called airtight, pressure bandages after surgical

5

removal of granulations on the distal extremities. Packs under these bandages are sometimes kept moist with dilute cresolic preparations.

Treatment of eumycotic mycetomas generally is unsatisfactory. If possible, the etiologic agent should be identified because actinomycotic mycetomas may be successfully treated with antibiotics and sulfonamides. See the treatment of actinomycosis and nocardiosis in Chapters 11 and 12.

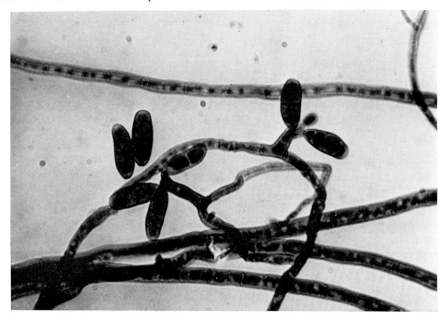

Fig. 4–7. Slide culture mount of *Curvularia geniculata.*

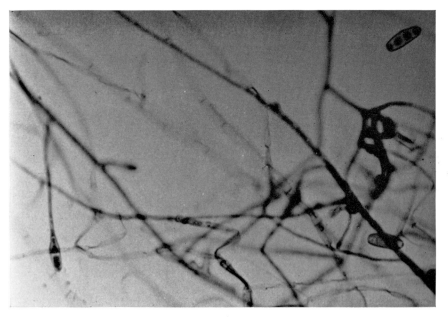

Fig. 4–8.   Spores of *Helminthosporium* species in culture.

REFERENCES

1. Annual Report of the Bureau of Animal Industry, 1893–94. Washington, U.S. Govt. Printing Office, 1896: 97–98.
2. Smith, F.: The Pathology of Bursatee. Vet. J., *19* (1884): 16–17.
3. de Haan, J. and Hoogkamer, L. J.: *Hyphomycosis destruens* equi, bosartige Schimmelkrankheit des Pferdes. Arch. f. Wissensch. u. Prakt. Tierheilk., Berl. *29* (1903): 395–410.
4. Van Overeem, C.: Beitrage zur Pilzflora von Niederlandisch Indien. 10. Ueber ein merkwurdiges Vorkommen von *Basidiobolus ranarum* Eidam. Bull. Jardin Bot., *7* (1925): 423–431.
5. Ajello, L., Georg, L. K., Kaplan, W. and Kaufman, L.: *Laboratory Manual for Medical Mycology*. Washington, U.S. Govt. Printing Office, 1963.
6. Tscherniak, W. S.: Zur Lehre von den bronchound pneumonomykosen der pferde. Arch. Wiss. Prakt. Tierheilk, *57* (1928): 417–444.
7. Bridges, C. H. and Emmons, C. W.: A Phycomycosis of Horses Caused by *Hyphomyces*. J. Amer. Vet. Med. Ass., *138* (1961): 579–589.
8. Bridges, C. H., Romane, W. M. and Emmons, C. W.: Phycomycosis of Horses Caused by *Entomophthora coronata*. J. Amer. Vet. Med. Ass., *140* (1962): 672–677.
9. Emmons C. W. and Bridges, C. H.: *Entomophthora coronata*, The Etiologic Agent of a Phycomycosis of Horses. Mycologia, *53* (1961): 307–312.
10. Bridges, C. H. as quoted in Bone, J. F., Ed.: *Equine Medicine and Surgery*. 1st edition, Santa Barbara, American Veterinary Publ., Inc., 1963.
11. Platt, K. B.: Institute of Tropical Veterinary Medicine, personal communication, 1970.
12. Rivolta, G.: Anat-physiol. Patol. Anim. (1885) as cited by Christiansen, M.: Mucormykose beim Schwein. I. Mitteilung. Virchows Arch., *273* (1929): 829–858.
13. Gleiser, C. A.: Mucormycosis in Animals. J. Amer. Vet. Med. Ass., *123* (1953): 441–445.
14. Howard, E. B.: Acute Mycotic Gastritis in a Dog. V.M./S.A.C., *61* (1966): 549–552.
15. Dawson, C. O., Wright, N. G., Aitken, J. O., Stevenson, S. H. and Gilbert, R. G.: Canine Phycomycosis: A Case Report. Vet. Rec., *84* (1969): 633–634.
16. Lucke, V. M., Morgan, D. G., English, M. P. and Endacott, G. M.: Phycomycosis in a Dog. Vet. Rec., *84* (1969): 645–646.
17. Heller, R. A., Hobson, H. P., Gowing, G. M., Storts, R. W., Read, W. K. and Bridges, C. H.: Three Cases of Phycomycosis in Dogs. V.M./S.A.C., *66* (1971): 472–476.
18. Jungherr, E.: Mycotic Affections of the Bovine Reproducitve System. J. Amer. Vet. Med. Ass., *39* (1935): 64–75.
19. Davis, C. L., Anderson, W. A. and McCrory, B. R.: Mucormycosis in Food-Producing Animals. J. Amer. Med. Vet. Ass., *126* (1955): 261–267.
20. Gitter, M. and Austwick, P. K. C.: The Presence of Fungi in Abomasal Ulcers of Young Calves: A Report of Seven Cases. Vet. Rec., *79* (1957): 924–928.
21. Cordes, D. O. and Shortridge, E. H.: Systemic Phycomycosis and Aspergillosis of Cattle. New Zeal. Vet. J., *16* (1968): 65–80.
22. Martin, J. E., Kroe, D. J., Bostrom, R. E., Johnson, D. J. and Whitney, R. A.: Rhino-Orbital Phycomycosis in a Rhesus Monkey (*Macaca mulatta*). J. Amer. Vet. Med. Ass., *155* (1969): 1253–1257.
23. Hessler, J. R., Woodard, J. C., Beattie, R. J. and Moreland, A. F.: Mucormycosis in a Rhesus Monkey. J. Amer. Vet. Med. Ass., *151* (1967): 909–913.
24. Kaplan, W., Goss, L. J., Ajello, L. and Ivens, M. S.: Pulmonary Mucormycosis in a Harp Seal Caused by *Mucor pusillus*. Mycopathologia, *12* (1960): 101–110.
25. Conant, N. F. et al.: *Manual of Clinical Mycology*. Philadelphia, W. B. Saunders Company, 1944.
26. Dodge, C. W.: *Medical Mycology*. St. Louis, C. V. Mosby Company, 1935: 110.
27. Bell, R. R.: Department of Veterinary Parasitology, Texas A&M Univ., College Station, personal communication, 1970.
28. Dikmans, G.: Check List of the Internal and External Animal Parasites of Domestic Animals in North America. Amer. J. Vet. Res., *6* (1945): 211–241.
29. Bridges, C. H.: Maduromycotic Mycetomas in Animals: *Curvularia geniculata* as an Etiologic Agent. Amer. J. Path., *33* (1957): 411–427.

30. Brodey, R. S., Schryver, H. F., Deubler, M. J., Kaplan, W. and Ajello, L.: Mycetoma in a Dog. J. Amer. Vet. Med. Ass., *151* (1967): 442–451.
31. Kurtz, H. J., Finco, D. R. and Perman, V.: Maduromycosis (*Allescheria boydii*) in a Dog. J. Amer. Vet. Med. Ass., *157* (1970): 917–921.
32. Jang, S. S. and Popp, J. A.: Eumycotic Mycetoma in a Dog Caused by *Allescheria boydii*. J. Amer. Vet. Med. Ass., *157* (1970): 1071–1076.
33. Bridges, C. H.: Maduromycosis of Bovine Nasal Mucosa (Nasal Granuloma of Cattle). Cornell Vet., *50* (1960): 469–484.
34. Roberts, E. D., McDaniel, H. A. and Carbey, E. A.: Maduromycosis of the Bovine Nasal Mucosa. J. Amer. Vet. Med. Ass., *142* (1963): 42–48.

CHAPTER | # Candidiasis

Candidiasis, caused by species of the genus *Candida* (usually *C. albicans*), is a sporadic disease of the alimentary canal of poultry sometimes having a high mortality rate. Predisposing factors are important in establishing infections. Swine are occasionally affected, sometimes with skin involvement. The disease may cause mastitis or abortion in cattle. Infections are rare in dogs, cats and horses.

HISTORY, GEOGRAPHIC DISTRIBUTION AND PREVALENCE

Infections caused by yeastlike fungi have been known in man for over 100 years. Lagenbeck, in 1839, first demonstrated a yeastlike fungus in the lesions of thrush. His finding was confirmed by Gruby in 1842, and the causative organism was named *Oidium albicans* by Robin in 1843.[1] Zopf named the fungus *Monilia albicans* in 1890, and for many years the disease was known as moniliasis. However, *Monilia* had originally been used for a different group of fungi, and although the use of the name moniliasis tends to persist in literature, it should be discontinued. Berkhout renamed the organism *Candida albicans* in 1923 and the disease, therefore, should be called candidiasis. In the United Kingdom, the name candidosis is generally used.

Candidiasis has been recognized in lower animals for over 50 years; however, other than in poultry, the early data regarding animal infections is scanty and often unsatisfactory.[2] Eberth reported candidiasis of chickens in 1858.[3] In 1932, Gierke reported an outbreak which caused 8 to 20 percent mortality in turkey poults in California.[4] The following year Jungherr[5] reported the loss of several thousand chicks in a commercial hatchery.

Although candidiasis both in human infants and in poultry is commonly called thrush, there are marked differences in the disease in the two hosts as well as in the various lower animal species affected. Candidiasis in man occurs in a variety of clinical forms. Oral infection (thrush) is important in infants and is troublesome in the aged, especially when chronic disease causes malnutrition or other forms of lowered general resistance. It is frequently severe in diabetes and during long-term treatment with corticosteroids or orally administered antibiotics.[1] Other well-delineated clinical types of infection are frequently seen in man. These range from localized infections of the skin, nails and hair follicles to vulvovaginitis, endocarditis, pulmonary infections and occasionally fatal systemic disease. These are well-documented in recent texts.[1,6] Predisposing factors causing unusual susceptibility are very frequently associated with the disease in man. It has become universally popular to cite candidiasis when ascribing increased incidences of mycoses to antibiotic therapy and the use of immunosuppressant drugs. There are a multitude of references which were largely summarized recently by Symers[7] who discussed the role of broad-spectrum antibiotics in altering the intestinal flora.

Several references have recently been cited which incriminate antibiotics as causes of dissemination of mycotic diseases, and the promiscuous use of antibiotics has been implicated as a contributing factor to the recent increase in mycotic infections in domestic animals.[8] The veterinary aspects of this problem, particularly with regard to poultry, need a careful evaluation. During the past 20 years, commercial animal feeds, especially those for poultry, have been "fortified" with antibiotics and/or residues. Indeed, often it is difficult to purchase rations free of these substances. Yet during this period there has not been an appreciable increase of candidiasis in poultry. Granted, the level of antibiotics present in feeds is quite low—low enough in fact that the normal intestinal flora may rapidly adjust to their presence and become resistant.

It is generally accepted that *Candida* species may be included with the typical intestinal flora, for the organisms can be isolated frequently from the feces or gastrointestinal tract of normal birds, man and lower animals. It is generally accepted, also, that predisposing factors are necessary to induce candidiasis in poultry. Antibiotics may be getting unjust blame that should be credited to such factors as avitaminosis, other nutritional disorders, bacterial or viral opportunists, and to poor management or housing practices.

Mills and Hirth[8] have reported systemic candidiasis in young calves on prolonged antibiotic therapy. Among the theories supporting antibiotic enhancement of candidial growth are: (1) direct stimulation of the fungus; (2) removal of organisms competing for nutrients; and (3) removal of organisms secreting antifungal substances. Of greater importance, Mills and Hirth believe, are the possible damage to tissues by the offending antibiotics, the conversion of *Candida* spp. to a more invasive form, the toxic products elaborated by *Candida* spp. and the depression of host responses to the infection.

The same authors stated that tissue damage by antibiotics may facilitate local invasion by *Candida* spp., and destruction of alimentary flora may cause a vitamin deficiency, thereby lowering resistance of tissues to invasion by *C. albicans*. Also, the organism flourishes when the antibiotic is tetracycline, since *C. albicans* utilizes this drug as a source of nitrogen. Further, the fungus produces an enzyme, leucine aminopeptidase which, by causing local tissue damage, may assist in establishing infection.[9]

Reports of candidiasis in swine have appeared frequently in recent years. As in poultry, the porcine infections occur most often in the very young. Various predisposing factors have been suspected including unthriftiness, antibiotic residues and other dietary factors including feeds high in glucose and maltose.

Fatal oral candidiasis of suckling pigs was reported by Kovalev[10] in 1947. Quin, in 1952, first associated antibiotic residues with mortality in pigs due to *Candida* spp.[11] McCrea and Osborne,[12] in 1957, and Gitter and Austwick the following year,[13] reported oral candidiasis in pigs. In the latter instance, the disease was associated with gastric mucormycosis. More recent reports have shown *Candida* spp. to have a predilection for the esophageal region of the gastric mucosa and the lower portion of the esophagus. Baker and Cadman identified *C. albicans* as the cause of disease in unthrifty pigs,[14] and Smith found *C. albicans* and *C. slooffii* both alone and in combination in pigs in New Zealand.[15] In a subsequent publication he concluded that the yeasts were secondary invaders only and that diet was responsible for the initial lesions.[16] *C. slooffii* has been isolated from pigs in England also but was not considered to be pathogenic.[17] Recently, Stedham and associates[18] have investigated the possible role of *C. albicans* in gastric ulcers in swine.

In almost all reported cases, porcine candidiasis has affected the oral, esophageal or gastric mucosa. In 1968, cutaneous candidiasis was described in 180 of a group of 450 garbage-fed swine.[19] No deaths occurred but the packer complained that the hams had to be skinned prior to their use for food.

As has previously been stated, *Candida* spp. can frequently—almost routinely—be isolated from the feces of normal birds and animals. It is interesting that in intestinal flora studies, *Candida* spp. often appear in the feces of normal pigs during the second week of life. This has been observed also in specific-pathogen free (SPF) pigs that were caesarian-obtained and barrier-maintained, and fed sterilized rations. Preliminary studies indicate that the flora which is established initially may prevail throughout life, and this may account for the presence or absence of yeasts in normal individuals.

Systemic bovine candidiasis was first reported in feed-lot cattle by McCarty in 1956.[20] More than a decade elapsed before Mills and Hirth reported systemic infections in calves.[8] The use of antibiotics was incriminated as a predisposing factor in both instances. During that decade, relatively few cases of bovine abortion were attributed to members of the genus *Candida*. Austwick and fellow workers[17] have recently reviewed what they consider to be valid cases, and their work indicates that—in addition to *C. albicans*—*C. tropicalis*, *C. krusei* and *C. parapsilosis* may occasionally have causal roles in bovine abortion. Smith has recently isolated *C. parapsilosis* from an aborted fetus and placenta.[15]

Evidence is gradually accumulating that *Candida* spp. other than *C. albicans* have pathogenic potential for animals. Predisposing factors are probably equally or more important for them. The student is cautioned that these species frequently inhabit the skin or alimentary tract of healthy animals, and that other more common etiologic agents must be considered and eliminated before making a diagnosis of candidiasis. It is important that tissue invasion be demonstrated also.

Surprisingly few cases of bovine mastitis due to *C. albicans* have been recorded. Stuart[21] isolated *Candida* spp. during an outbreak which followed infusion of udders with penicillin. Prasad and Prasad[22] identified *C. parapsilosis* in mastitic milk following antibiotic therapy for a preexisting bacterial infection. Austwick et al.[17] examined 90 cultures of milk samples and, among the yeasts isolated, found *Candida* spp. to predominate. *C. krusei* and *C. tropicalis* were the most frequent isolates. Information on the possible role of antibiotic therapy and preexisting infections was not presented.

Equine candidiasis is quite rare and apparently has been described only as a secondary infection. Tatezawa[23] has reported endometritis in mares, and Collins[24] indicates finding *Candida* spp. associated with cervical and uterine infections. In both reports, the infections were considered to be secondary and related to anti-biotic therapy.

Feline candidiasis is equally rare and a primary etiologic role for *Candida* spp. has not been established. Schiefer and Weis[25] have reported finding *Candida* spp. on the surface of granulation tissue in the intestinal mucosa. Two other cases they reported were associated with panleucopenia and antibiotic therapy.[26] Austwick and coworkers[17] have reported a single isolation of *C. tropicalis* from feline intestine.

The first reported case of canine candidiasis has unusual interest for veterinarians. In 1949, Reich and Nechtow[27] reported that dogs with genital *C. albicans* infection were the source of reinfection for a human female. The dogs, male and female with balanoposthitis and vaginitis respectively, slept under the covers with the lady and, on occasion, voided in the bathtub where she bathed. It is now apparent that canine candidiasis is quite rare and, to our knowledge, no other reports of canine genital infections are recorded. In retrospect, this may have been a case of human-to-animal transmission.

Cutaneous candidiasis in dogs is rare. Král and Uscavage[28] described a case with lesions over much of the skin area which developed following a long period of oral and parenteral antibiotic therapy. Král and Schwartzman[29] reported seeing three other cases, but they were not described. Schwartzman and associates[30] have induced cutaneous *C. albicans* infections experimentally in dogs. The lesion resembled that of pyo-traumatic dermatitis (hotspot).

Canine otitis, primarily caused by *Candida* spp., may be nonexistent. Many isolations have been made, and cases have been reported,[17] but it is doubted that these fungi are ever the initial pathogens. Fraser[31] has reported three cases of acute mycotic otitis, one of which was caused by *C. albicans* and the other two by *C. tropicalis*. All were encountered in animals which had received prolonged anti-biotic therapy. The *C. tropicalis* infections were secondary to otitis associated with coagulase-positive staphylococci, the other was secondary to a *Pseudomonas aeruginosa* infection.

If the criterion of primary invasion by a fungus is applied, the authors believe that animal otomycosis rarely, if ever, occurs. Several other fungi have been associated with otitis in man and animals, particularly members of the genus *Pityrosporum*. In one instance, otitis resulted from instilling a culture of *Pityrosporum* sp. in the ear. However, in view of the fact that canine otitis can result from applications of sterile distilled water, experimental fungal infections of the canine ear have questionable value.

Poultry pathologists and researchers are not in complete agreement regarding the significance of candidiasis (thrush, mycosis of the digestive tract) in poultry. Some authorities minimize its importance, and it has been deleted from some instruction manuals and many general discussions of poultry diseases. In certain limited geographic areas and in some diagnostic laboratories, the disease rates a higher order of importance. There is general agreement that poor management and unsani-tary conditions are important predisposing factors and that the disease is more severe in poults than in chicks. Candidiasis is apparently more troublesome to gamebird producers than to commercial poultry operators. The former are often hobbyists with inadequate knowledge of good sanitation and management practices.

In recent years, reports of outbreaks of candidiasis in poultry have appeared infrequently. Austwick and co-workers[17] have recently reviewed aspects of the

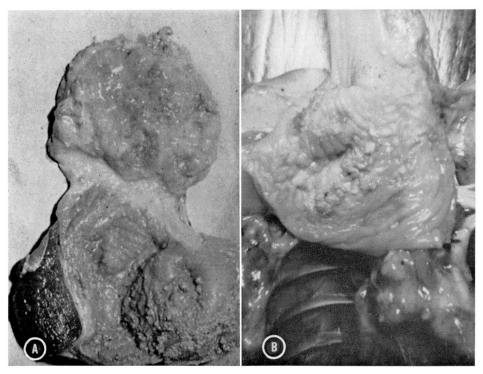

Fig. 5-1.   **A.** Lesions in proventriculus and gizzard of poult with *Candida albicans* infection. **B.** Candidiasis of crop.

disease in England.   The effects of vitamin A deficiency and high-level chlortetracycline on experimental candidiasis of turkeys have been studied by Tripathy and associates,[45] and the role of essential fatty acid deficiency in *C. albicans* infection in the chick has been reported by Wagstaff and colleagues.[32]

Many European workers believe that *C. albicans*, *Candida* spp. or other yeastlike fungi have a primary etiologic role in avian infectious enterohepatitis (blackhead). Their contention is in almost direct opposition to the belief of Anglo-American researchers who recognize the protozoan *Histomonas meleagridis* as the primary etiologic agent.   Kemp and Reid evaluated the role of *C. albicans* and *H. meleagridis* in production of the disease in the United States and they did not isolate *C. albicans* from any field cases but commonly recovered *H. meleagridis*.   Although *C. albicans* was often observed to be present in the digestive tract, it was not isolated from livers of natural cases of blackhead in turkeys nor could it be recovered following experimental inoculations with *C. albicans* by oral, rectal, intravenous or cecal wall inoculation.[33]   In another study, Reid and associates[34] obtained tissues and fungus cultures from European workers and succeeded in reproducing the disease syndrome only when suitable bacteria were present also.   Their experiments indicate that a dual etiology is involved—*H. meleagridis* and at least one species of bacteria (*Escherichia coli*, *Clostridium perfringens* or others).

Candidiasis apparently has no geographic limitations.   *Candida* spp. are present with man, animals and birds wherever they reside, and they require only the opportunity to become invasive. Animal cases, and particularly those of birds, are no doubt much more frequent than reports indicate.

CLINICAL SIGNS AND PATHOLOGY

Due to various predisposing factors and related pathologic conditions, the clinical signs of candidiasis in poultry are not specific. Affected chicks may show unsatisfactory growth, a stunted appearance, listlessness and roughness of the feathers.[35] Common clinical signs in poults are listlessness, loss of appetite, tendency to stand around with heads drawn back on the shoulders and a sunken appearance of the chest. The eyes and sinuses appear sunken and the heads haggard.[36]

In avian candidiasis, the gross lesions are usually confined to the crop. Less frequently, the fungus may invade the mouth, infraorbital sinuses, esophagus, proventriculus, gizzard and intestines. The mucosa of the crop is thickened with circular, whitish, raised ulcerlike lesions, often with a scaly appearing surface. The lesions have been described as having a "turkish-towel-like" or "curdy" appearance and are easily removed from the surface.[36] In both acute and mild cases, the crop surface may show a catarrhal to mucoid exudate with a tendency to form a pseudomembrane. Mouth and esophageal lesions may appear as ulcerlike patches.

Histologically, extensive destruction of the stratified epithelium may occur deep in the malpighian layer. Many lesions are characterized by the absence of inflammatory reaction, and walled-off ulcers or extensive diphtheroid to diphtheric membranes may be observed.[5]

Clinical signs in calves include watery diarrhea and melena with subsequent anorexia and dehydration, and gradual progression to prostration and death.

Bovine mammary infections caused by *Candida* spp. are often mild and transient; some are self-limiting. The more severe infections have followed antibiotic infusions. *C. tropicalis* was incriminated in one outbreak in which all treated animals developed acute mastitis with varying degrees of severity. The udders developed extensive swelling of a spongy consistency. Milk from the affected quarters was grey and viscid. Body temperatures of some cows ranged from 104° to 107° F. Some individuals were anorectic and lame, and milk production was drastically decreased.[37]

Candidiasis of swine has been reported most frequently in piglets. Vomition, diarrhea and emaciation are the most consistent clinical signs. Concomitance with other disorders, particularly unthriftiness and metabolic disease, is the general rule.

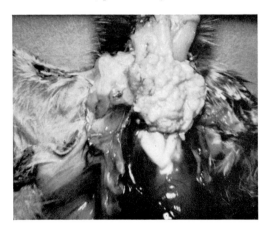

Fig. 5–2. Crop mycosis (C. *albicans*) in turkey poult.

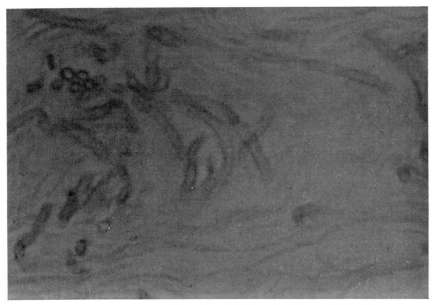

Fig. 5–3.   Avian crop mycosis.   The mycelial or M form of C. *albicans* may be
seen in the mucosa.

Baker and Cadman have questioned whether *C. albicans* is capable of infecting
normal pigs.[14] However, a recent investigation of stomach lesions in market-aged
swine by Kadel and co-workers[38] indicated a relationship of *Candida* spp. to
altered keratinization and ulceration.   Histologically, the lesions varied from slight
erosive changes of the stratum corneum to true ulceration, lymphofollicular hyperplasia, neutrophilic and eosinophilic infiltration, thrombosis and edema.

LABORATORY DIAGNOSIS

The diagnosis of candidiasis requires more than the isolation and identification of
Candida species, and a diagnosis of candidiasis should never appear on a laboratory
report. This is especially applicable when a member of the genus other than *C. albicans* is identified. Unlike many of the fungus pathogens which are considered
etiologic agents of disease by virtue of their presence in clinical materials, *Candida*
spp. are commonly present as harmless commensals at the site of lesions.   The
laboratory is confined to the role of identifying a potential pathogen; interpretation
and diagnosis should be reserved for the clinician.

Direct Microscopic Examination

Skin scrapings are examined in 10 percent KOH mounts. Mucosal scrapings may
be smeared on slides for Gram staining or direct mounts may be examined in
lactophenol cotton blue.   Rounded or oval budding cells, 3–6 μ in diameter, and
fragments of mycelium, sometimes with budding cells attached, may be demonstrated. If both blastospores (budding, yeastlike or Y forms) and pseudohyphae*

---

* Pseudohyphae are a type of mycelium formed by blastospores that remain attached after
budding to form chains of elongated cells. Such "mycelium" shows indentations at the
septae between the cells in the chains, and frequently secondary budding at these points.

or true mycelium* (mycelial or M-forms) are found, a presumptive diagnosis of candidiasis may be made since the presence of both the Y and M forms usually indicates invasion of the tissue by *Candida* species.

Culture

Since most submissions from animals are obtained at sites normally inhabited by bacteria (e.g. mouth, esophagus, crop, stomach or skin), it is essential that selective media be used for primary isolation. Sabouraud dextrose broth and Sabouraud agar adequately support growth of *Candida* spp. and restrict the growth of many bacteria. Satisfactory growth is obtained with most strains at either room temperature or 37° C. *C. albicans* is not inhibited by antibacterial antibiotics or cycloheximide, and isolation media containing these antibiotics is helpful. Some *Candida* spp., however—particularly *C. parapsilosis*, *C. krusei* and some strains of *C. tropicalis*—are sensitive to cycloheximide, therefore media free of antibiotics should be used in parallel.

If bacterial contaminants occur, they can usually be eliminated by inoculating yeastlike cultures to four tubes of Sabouraud dextrose broth to which have been added: one drop, two drops, three drops and four drops of 1N HCl, respectively. Incubate at 37° C. overnight. Subculture from the acid tube that is free of bacteria (generally the tube containing two or three drops of acid) to a blood agar plate at 37° C. Colonies are then picked from this plate and subcultured to Sabouraud dextrose agar.[39]

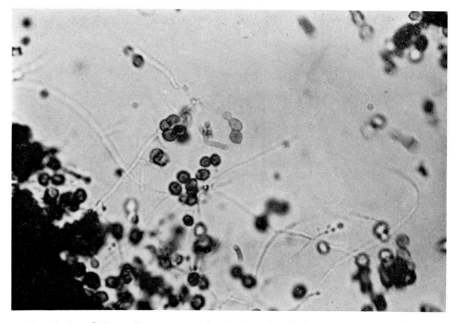

Fig. 5–4. Chlamydospore production by C. *albicans* on cornmeal agar.

---

* True mycelium is also formed under certain conditions. This is formed by the extension of a germ tube from a blastospore to produce a parallel-sided filament. This secondarily forms septations by concentric invagination of the cell wall.

On Sabouraud agar, young colonies of *Candida albicans* are white, soft and usually smooth. Old colonies often have submerged mycelial growth at their margins that has a feathery appearance.

Microscopic examination reveals round, oval and budding cells. In old cultures, pseudohyphae and occasionally true mycelium may be observed, particularly if submerged growth at the margin of the colony is examined. This latter observation is characteristic of the genus.

The production of characteristic chlamydospores on cornmeal agar is a widely used and highly specific method for the identification of *Candida albicans*. Surface spread of the growth and spore production is enhanced by the addition of one-percent Tween 80 to the medium. The organism to be tested should be scratched into the surface of the agar with the inoculating needle held at about a 45-degree angle. It is important that the inoculum be taken from a very dilute suspension of the culture in question. Part of the inoculated area should be covered with a flame-sterilized coverslip. The plates are incubated at room temperature for 48 hours and, if characteristic growth is not apparent, reincubated for two or three days longer. Known cultures can be streaked into the same plates used for the unknown being tested. Slide mounts of submerged growth at the edge of the streaks, both outside and from under the coverslip, are examined for development of mycelium and chlamydospores. If the characteristic chlamydospores develop, this is adequate for the identification of *C. albicans*. Absolute specificity of the test is prevented by possible errors of interpretation due to similar, although morphologically different, rare chlamydospore production by other *Candida* spp., especially *C. guilliermondi* and *C. stellatoidea*.*

Another identification test with at least equal specificity has had wide acceptance in recent years. This is the "serum tube" test (filamentation test) introduced by Taschdjian and colleagues.[40] It is based on the production of filamentous outgrowths (pseudo-germ tubes/pseudomycelium) by cells of *C. albicans* when inoculated into serum and incubated at 37° C. for one to two hours. The test has many advantages. It is fast, simple, quite specific and does not require the use of pure

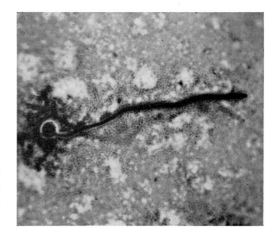

Fig. 5–5. Filamentous pseudo-germ tube/pseudomycelium produced by *C. albicans* in serum medium.

* *C. stellatoidea* is closely related to *C. albicans* and is considered by some writers to be a variant of this species.

TABLE 5-1. Candida Identification Chart*

Species	Morphology on Corn Meal Agar Cut-streak plate	Sabouraud dextrose broth Growth characteristics	Sugar* fermentation reactions				Sugar Assimilation						
			D	M	S	L	Dextrose	Galactose	Lactose	Maltose	Raffinose	Sucrose	Cellobiose
C. albicans	Irregular or spherical clusters of blastospores of septa. Chlamydospores single or in clusters. May be very numerous (chlamydospores do not develop at 37° C.)	No surface growth	Ag	Ag	A or O	O	+	+	O	+	O	+	O
C. guilliermondii	Very fine mycelium. Small clusters of blastospores at the septa.	No surface growth	O or Ag	O	O or Ag	O	+	+	O	+	+	+	+
C. krusei	Elongate cells forming a branched mycelium easily disintegrated. "Crossed sticks" at septa.	Wide surface film	Ag	O	O	O	+	O	O	O	O	O	O
C. parapsilosis	Fine and coarse mycelium (giant forms). Blastospores single or in short chains at septa or distal ends of cells.	No surface growth	Ag or A	O or A	O or A	O	+	+	O	+	O	+	+
C. pseudotropicalis	Very elongate cells which readily fall apart and lie parallel. "Logs in stream"	No surface growth	Ag	O	Ag	Ag	+	+	+	O	+	+	+ or O
C. stellatoidea (probably a variant of C. albicans).	More extensive mycelium with irregular or spherical clusters of blastospores at septa. Chlamydospores rare (may show a supporting cell).	No surface growth	Ag	Ag	A or O	O	+	+	O	+	O	O	O
C. tropicalis	Blastospores anywhere along mycelium or in irregular clusters. Chlamydospores very rare.	Narrow surface film with bubbles	Ag	Ag	Ag	O	+	+	O	+	O	+	+ or O

* D = dextrose M = maltose S = sucrose L = lactose

* From Ajello, L. et al., CDC Laboratory Manual for Medical Mycology, Washington, U.S. Dept. of Health, Education and Welfare, Public Health Service.

cultures. It does not, however, differentiate *C. albicans* from *C. stellatoidea*. A modification, using egg white instead of serum, has been described by Buckley and van Uden.[41]

Selective media for the isolation of *Candida* spp., which are designed to differentiate species by variation of colony coloring, have been found useful in some laboratories. The agar medium of Pagano and fellow workers[42] utilizes neomycin to inhibit bacteria and tetrazolium as a color marker. *C. albicans* grows as a cream to light pink colored colony. Other *Candida* spp. vary from white to deep red; other yeasts, however, are not entirely inhibited and a presumptive identification only can be made. However, some workers find the medium useful only for primary selection of isolates for further study.

Because of the simplicity and specificity of the chlamydospore and serum tube tests, *C. albicans* may be quickly identified with confidence with a combination of these two tests. Confirmation may be obtained with sugar fermentation and assimilation tests. These latter tests and other growth characteristics are required for identification of other pathogenic *Candida* spp. (Table 5–1). Detailed methodology for sugar fermentation and assimilation tests for yeasts and yeastlike organisms may be found in standard texts.[46,47]

Pure cultures are a critical prerequisite for fermentation and assimilation tests and, in addition, the isolate being tested should be serially transferred at least three times on a sugar-free medium. Fermentation tubes should be topped with melted vaseline. Incubate at 37° C. for 10 days.

Pathogenicity Tests

Both rabbits and mice succumb to intravenous inoculation of *C. albicans*, but there is no practical use for the test since other *Candida* spp. may cause death in these animals also.

Immunology

There are no dependable serologic tests for the diagnosis of candidiasis of animals.

DIFFERENTIAL DIAGNOSIS

Avian candidiasis must be differentiated from pox, trichomoniasis of the upper digestive tract and histomoniasis. Differential staining techniques for diagnosis of histomoniasis and mycosis in poultry have been evaluated recently by Kemp and Reid.[43]

In differential diagnosis of porcine cutaneous candidiasis, the infection must be distinguished from mange, ringworm and parakeratosis.[19] Cutaneous candidiasis in dogs may resemble pyo-traumatic dermatitis; disseminated infection may resemble geotrichosis, a mycotic disease considered to be rare in animals and man. Lincoln and Adcock[48] recently described a canine case, and their report includes an excellent literature review (for man and animals). As a general rule, cutaneous and mucosal lesions of candidiasis in all animal species must be differentiated from bacterial infections and dermatophytosis.

EPIDEMIOLOGY

Candida spp. are so commonly present in the gastrointestinal tract of man and animals and have been found so infrequently in nature that it seems proper to consider the diseases they cause as endogenous in origin. In certain circumstances in man, individual to individual transmission occurs. Balanoposthitis has resulted from vaginal contact, and there is a mother to child transmission at birth through the vagina. Similar transmission has not been reported in animals.

Maddy has suggested the possibility that fecal contamination of meat at slaughter serves as a source of animal-to-man transmission.[44] Fecal contamination of feed undoubtedly accounts for the spread of candidiasis in closely housed animals.

TREATMENT

The majority of cases of candidiasis in animals are associated with predisposing disease, unsanitary conditions or with prior medication with antibacterial antibiotics. Correction of these conditions is the first step in therapy. Oral, cutaneous and aural lesions may respond favorably to nystatin ointment, topical applications of amphotericin B or one-percent iodine.

Avian candidiasis is also predisposed by the conditions mentioned above. Therefore a fair appraisal of the therapeutic value of a given drug in field outbreaks is difficult. Copper sulfate, at 1:2000 dilution in drinking water, has been regarded as an effective treatment. Some workers consider it to be ineffective as a prophylactic or treatment.[49] Mayeda[50] recorded favorable results with copper sulfate, quaternary ammonium compounds and nystatin provided strict conditions for use were met. Segregation of affected birds and maintenance of a clean water supply are essential prerequisites to successful therapy. For reasons of economy and because of past results, poultry veterinarians in the Texas diagnostic laboratories routinely recommend treatment with copper sulfate in the drinking water (one pound in 100 gallons plus one gallon of vinegar). Some recommend changing to nystatin if copper sulfate is not effective.

Recently Wood[51] has reported on the control of candidiasis in hand-reared partridges with dilute formic acid applied as a spray on the feed.

REFERENCES

1. Wilson, J. W. and Plunkett, O. A.: *The Fungous Diseases of Man.* Berkeley, University of California Press, 1965.
2. Ainsworth, G. C. and Austwick, P. K. C.: *Fungal Diseases of Animals.* Farnham Royal, Bucks, England, Commonwealth Agricultural Bureaux, 1959.
3. Eberth, J.: Einige Beobachtungen von Pflanzlichen Parasiten bei Thieren-Arch. f. Path. Anat. u. Physiol., *39* (1858): 522.
4. Gierke, A. G.: A Preliminary Report on a Mycosis of Turkeys. Bull. Cal. Dept. Agri., *21* (1932): 229–231.
5. Jungherr, E. L.: Observations on a Severe Outbreak of Mycosis in Chicks. J. Agri. Res., *46* (1933): 169–178.
6. Emmons, C. W., Binford, C. H. and Utz, J. P.: *Medical Mycology.* 2nd edition, Philadelphia, Lea & Febiger, 1970.
7. Symers, W. St. C.: in Winner, H. I. and Hurley, E. Eds.: *Symposium on Candida Infections.* London, E & S Livingstone Ltd., 1966.
8. Mills, J. H. L. and Hirth, R. S.: Systemic Candidiasis in Calves on Prolonged Antibiotic Therapy. J. Amer. Vet. Med. Ass., *150* (1967): 862–870.
9. Kim, V. P., Adachi, K., and Chow, D.: Leucine Aminopeptidase in *Candida albicans.* J. Invest. Derm., *38* (1962): 115–116.
10. Kovalev, A. A.: Mycotic Aphthous Stomatitis in Suckling Pigs. Veterinariia, *24* (1947): 18.

11. Quin, A. H.: Newer Problems in Swine Diseases—Control and Treatment. Canad. J. Comp. Med., *16* (1952): 265–270.

12. McCrea, M. R. and Osborne, A. D.: A Case of Thrush (Candidiasis) in a Piglet. J. Comp. Path. Ther., *67* (1957): 343–344.

13. Gitter, M. and Austwick, P. K. C.: Mucormycosis and Moniliasis in a Litter of Suckling Pigs. Vet. Rec., *71* (1959): 6–11.

14. Baker, E. D. and Cadman, L. P.: Candidiasis in Pigs in Northwestern Wisconsin. J. Amer. Vet. Med. Ass., *142* (1963): 763–767.

15. Smith, J. M. B.: Candidiasis in Animals in New Zealand. Sabouraudia, *5* (1967): 220–225.

16. Smith, J. M. B.: Animal Mycoses in New Zealand. Mycopathologia, *34* (1968): 323–336.

17. Austwick, P. K. C., Pepin, G. A., Thompson, J. C. and Yarrow, D.: in Winner, H. I. and Hurley, R., Eds.: *Symposium on Candida Infections.* London, E & S Livingstone Ltd., 1966.

18. Stedham, M. A., Kelley, D. C. and Coles, E. H.: Influence of Dietary Sugar on Growth of *Candida albicans* in the Porcine Digestive Tract and Lesions in the Esophageal Area of the Stomach. Amer. J. Vet. Res., *28* (1967): 153–159.

19. Reynolds, I. M., Miner, P. W. and Smith, R. E.: Cutaneous Candidiasis in Swine. J. Amer. Vet. Med. Ass., *152* (1968): 182–186.

20. McCarty, R. T.: Moniliasis as a Systemic Infection in Cattle: Field Case Reports. Vet. Med., *51* (1956): 562–564.

21. Stuart, P.: An Outbreak of Bovine Mastitis from which Yeasts were Isolated and Attempts to Reproduce the Conditions Experimentally. Vet. Rec., *63* (1951): 314.

22. Prasad, L. B. M. and Prasad, S.: Bovine Mastitis Caused by a Yeast in India. Vet. Rec., *79* (1966): 809–810.

23. Tatezawa, E.: Uterine Candiosis in Mares. Jap. J. Vet. Sci., *20* (1958): 299.

24. Collins, S. M.: A Study of the Incidence of Cervical and Uterine Infection in Thoroughbred Mares in Ireland. Vet. Rec., *76* (1964): 673–674.

25. Schiefer, Von B. and Weis, E.: Zur Histopathologic der durch Candida-Aspergillus-und Mucor-Arten verursachten Darmmykosen bei Katzen mit Panleukopenie. Deutsche tieraztl. Wchnschr., *72* (1965): 73–76.

26. Schiefer, Von B. and Weis, E.: Soormykose des Darmes bei Katzen. Deutsche tieraztl. Wchnschr., *66* (1959): 275–277.

27. Reich, W. J. and Nechtow, M. J.: Canine Genital Moniliasis as a Source of Reinfection in the Human Female. JAMA, *141* (1949): 991–992.

28. Král, F. and Uscavage, J. P.: Cutaneous Candidiasis in a Dog. J. Amer. Vet. Med. Ass., *136* (1960): 612–615.

29. Král, F. and Schwartzman, R. M.: *Veterinary and Comparative Dermatology.* 2nd edition, J. B. Lippincott Company, Philadelphia, 1964.

30. Schwartzman, R. M., Deubler, M. J. and Dice II, P. F.: Experimentally Induced Cutaneous Moniliasis (*Candida albicans*) in the Dog. J. Small Anim. Pract., *8* (1965): 327–332.

31. Fraser, G.: The Fungal Flora of the Canine Ear. J. Comp. Path. Ther., *71* (1961): 1–5.

32. Wagstaff, R. K., Jensen, L. S., Tripathy, S. B. and Kenzy, S. G.: Essential Fatty Acid Deficiency and *Candida Albicans* Infection in the Chick. Avian Diseases, *12* (1968): 186–190.

33. Kemp, R. L. and Reid, W. M.: Studies on the Etiology of Blackhead Disease: The Roles of *Histomonas meleagridis* and *Candida albicans* in the United States. Poult. Sci., *45* (1966): 1296–1302.

34. Reid, W. M., Kemp, R. L. and Johnson, J.: Studies on the Comparative Roles of *Histomonas meleagridis* and *Candida albicans* in the Production of Blackhead in European Poultry. Zbl. Vet. Med., B, *14* (1967): 179–185.

35. Chute, H. L.: Diseases Caused by Fungi in Biester, H. E. and Schwarte, L. H., Eds.: *Diseases of Poultry.* 5th edition, Ames, Iowa State University Press, 1965.

36. Hinshaw, W. R.: Diseases of the Turkey in Biester, H. E. and Schwarte, L. H., Eds.: *Diseases of Poultry.* 5th edition, Ames, Iowa State University Press, 1965.

37. Loken, K. I., Thompson, E. S., Hoyt, H. H. and Ball, R. A.:   Infection of the Bovine Udder with *Candida tropicalis*. J. Amer. Vet. Med. Ass., *134* (1959): 401–403.

38. Kadel, W. L., Kelley, D. C. and Coles, E. H.:   Survey of Yeastlike Fungi and Tissue Changes in Esophagastric Region of Stomachs of Swine. Amer. J. Vet. Res., *30* (1969): 401–408.

39. Ajello, L., Georg, L. K., Kaplan, W. and Kaufman, L.:   *Laboratory Manual for Medical Mycology*. Pub. Health Serv. Pub. No. 994, Washington, U.S. Govt. Printing Office, 1963.

40. Taschdjian, C. L., Burchall, J. J. and Kozinn, P. J.:   Rapid Identification of *Candida albicans* by Filamentation on Serum and Serum Substitutes. J. Dis. Child., *99* (1960): 212–215.

41. Buckley, H. R. and van Uden, N.:   The Identification of *Candida albicans* within Two Hours by the Use of An Egg White Slide Preparation. Sabouraudia, *2* (1963): 205–208.

42. Pagano, J., Levin, J. D. and Trejo, W.:   Diagnostic Medium for Differentiation of Species of Candida. Antibiot. Ann., *12* (1958): 137–143.

43. Kemp, R. L. and Reid, W. M.:   Staining Techniques for Differential Diagnosis of Histomoniasis and Mycosis in Domestic Poultry. Avian Diseases, *10* (1966): 357–363.

44. Maddy, K. T.:   Epidemiology and Ecology of Deep Mycoses of Man and Animals. Arch. Derm., *96* (1967): 409–417.

45. Tripathy, S. B., Kenzy, S. G. and Mathey, W. J.:   Effects of Vitamin-A Deficiency and High-Level Chlortetracycline on Experimental Candidiasis of Turkeys. Avian Diseases, *11* (1967): 327–335.

46. Lodder, J. and Kreger-Van Rij, N.:   *The Yeasts: A Taxonomic Study*. Amsterdam, North Holland Publishing Co., 1952.

47. Fungal Infections (Chapter XXIV) in *APHA Diagnostic Procedures and Reagents*. 5th edition, New York, American Public Health Association, 1970.

48. Lincoln, S. D. and Adcock, J. L.:   Disseminated Geotrichosis in a Dog. Pathologia Vet., *5* (1968): 282–289.

49. Underwood, P. C., Collins, J. H., Durbin, C. G., Hodges, F. A. and Zimmerman, H. E. Jr.:   Critical Tests with Copper Sulfate for Experimental Moniliasis (Crop Mycosis) of Chickens and Turkeys. Poult. Sci., *35* (1956): 599–605.

50. Mayeda, B.:   Candiasis in Turkeys and Chickens in the Sacramento Valley of California. Avian Diseases, *5* (1961): 232–243.

51. Wood, N. A.:   The Control of Candidiasis (Moniliasis) in Partridges with Formic Acid. Vet. Rec., *84* (1969): 443.

CHAPTER **6** | Aspergillosis

Aspergillosis, caused by *Aspergillus fumigatus, Aspergillus flavus* and other *Aspergillus species,* is a disease primarily of respiratory tissues characterized by inflammatory granulomatous lesions. Hematogenous dissemination to other organs may occur. Occasionally the eye, skin, meninges and reproductive tract are invaded. The disease is relatively rare in domestic and pet animals but occurs frequently in avian species.

HISTORY, GEOGRAPHIC DISTRIBUTION AND PREVALENCE

Aspergillosis has been recognized as an avian disease since 1815 when it was reported in a jay by Mayer and Emmert.[1] By the end of the nineteenth century, diseases caused by members of the genus *Aspergillus* had been extensively studied, and almost all known forms of the disease in domestic animals and birds had been reported. Chute and coworkers[2] in 1962 published a bibliography of avian mycoses which listed over 700 references to fungi in birds. It is generally accepted that *Aspergillus fumigatus* is the most pathogenic member of the genus. *A. flavus* is quite important in captive birds also.[3] Various other *Aspergillus* spp. have pathogenic potential and occasionally are reported as causal agents of disease.

A tremendous volume of literature has appeared concerning the veterinary aspects of aspergillosis. An excellent review was presented by Ainsworth and Austwick[4] in 1959. The majority of cases they recorded in mammalian species occurred in the latter part of the nineteenth century and early in the twentieth century. In most other mycotic diseases, a marked increase of reports occurred around 1950 and shortly thereafter. Reports of aspergillosis in domestic and pet animals have appeared only sporadically in recent years.

Although equine aspergillosis was first disclosed over 100 years ago, the disease is apparently quite rare in horses. Most of the early reported cases involved the nasal sinuses as local infections. One case with meningeal involvement and another which developed rapidly into a generalized infection have been described.[4] Few cases have been described in recent literature, and this is somewhat surprising in view of the types of feed consumed by stabled horses. *Aspergillus fumigatus* has been associated with persistent diarrhea in colts.[5] Equine abortions may occasionally be caused by *Aspergillus* spp.[6,7]

Ovine aspergillosis occurs infrequently. Cases of pulmonary infection in lambs have been described in which *A. fumigatus* was recovered from all lung lesions.[8] Pure cultures of this organism were obtained from a lamb with a generalized infection.[9] Both the vascular and lymphatic systems appeared to be involved in the extension of the infection from the respiratory system to other organs in the body.

Several forms of bovine aspergillosis have been recorded, although infrequently. A mycotic granuloma in the skin of a cow from which *A. terreus* was subsequently isolated has been described by Davis and Schaefer.[10] *A. fumigatus* has been isolated from lung tissue of a six-week-old calf with disseminated mycotic pneumonia which resembled miliary tuberculosis.[11] Griffin[12] has described the clinical course, cultural and histopathologic findings in pulmonary aspergillosis of a three-week-old calf. A fatal case of pulmonary aspergillosis in a cow was described by Molello and Busey.[13]

Austwick[14] has found *Aspergillus fumigatus* in the lungs of apparently healthy cows during the course of experiments on mycotic abortion. Also this organism has been isolated from the placentae of cows that had aborted.[15]

In recent years, with the reduction in incidence of bovine brucellosis, mycotic abortions have an increased interest and importance. There is evidence that the incidence of mycotic abortions may be increasing. In one study, covering 189 bovine abortions due to various causes, 16.4 percent were mycotic.[16] *A. fumigatus* was isolated most frequently. Abortions caused by experimental inoculation of the organism have been studied in both cattle[17] and sheep.[18]

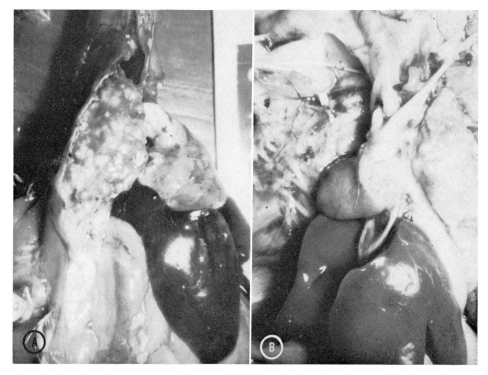

Fig. 6–1. **A.** Avian aspergillosis. Nodular lesions in lungs. Exudates in air sacs. **B.** Caseous exudate in air sacs. (Courtesy of Dr. S. E. Glass)

Porcine aspergillosis apparently is very rare. A few cases are recorded in early literature, but confirmatory cultural studies were not made in most instances.

Authentic cases of aspergillosis in dogs and cats are quite rare also. Apparently no cases of pulmonary or generalized infection in the dog have been described. Isolations have been made from ear and nasal infections, usually in combination with other organisms. Fatal pulmonary aspergillosis has been reported in cats.[19,20] The diagnoses were made on the basis of histopathologic studies. No culture or species identification attempts were reported.

Avian aspergillosis is common and is encountered in poultry in two main forms: (1) acute outbreaks with high morbidity and high mortality in young birds; and (2) in adult birds as a chronic condition affecting individual birds. It is more important in turkeys but may affect chickens also. The acute form is commonly called "brooder pneumonia" by poultrymen. Many species of the genus *Aspergillus* have been incriminated as the causative agents of respiratory disease in poultry, but *A. fumigatus* is the species most commonly encountered. *A. flavus* is quite important also, and in some studies has been the organism isolated most frequently.[21,22] Ostensibly the birds become infected by inhalation of spores which are present in feed, litter or in the soil of the premises. The disease can be experimentally produced by blowing spores into the trachea,[23] by feeding mash containing the spores[24] and by contaminating feed in a forced-draft incubator.[25]

Healthy birds can apparently withstand a moderate degree of exposure to spores. Individual cases that occur in adult flocks are attributed to predisposing disease or massive exposure.

Aspergillosis is usually considered to be a disease of captivity, but it is known to exist in freeliving wild birds. In one study, 17 of 18 cases were due to *A. fumigatus*.[26] Rosen has presented evidence that this disease may be epizootic in diving ducks and

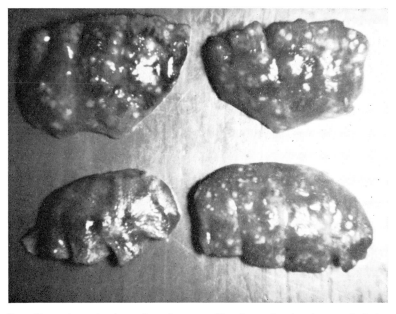

Fig. 6–2.   Granulomata in avian lungs.   The lung in the lower left is normal.
(Courtesy of Dr. S. E. Glass)

free-flying passerine birds, and that its occurrence is strongly influenced by the prevailing character of weather and climate.[27]

Penguins often have high mortality rates due to aspergillosis after they are transported to the confining environment of a zoo.[3]   Whether they are especially susceptible and become infected in captivity or have subclinical infections that become clinically apparent during transport and confinement is an unresolved question.

Aspergillus fumigatus has been reported to penetrate egg shells and infect embryos.[28] The fungus has been isolated from incubators in which chicks were hatched; they later developed pneumomycosis with high mortality.

The aspergilli are present as saprophytes in all climates, and the diseases they cause have a worldwide distribution. Aspergillosis has been reported in almost all species of domestic animals and birds and in many wild species.[4] Recently, the African okapi,[32] American alligator[33] and Japanese quail[34] have been added to the list of hosts.

CLINICAL SIGNS AND PATHOLOGY

In the acute form of the disease in young birds, the main signs are anorexia, sleepiness, gasping, and sometimes convulsions and death. The fungus occasionally invades the brain and causes paralysis or other signs of CNS involvement. Ocular infections occur commonly, usually unilaterally. The birds fail to grow and keep the affected eyes closed; later some develop cheesy exudates in the conjunctival sacs. The chronic form affects older birds, often only a single individual or a few birds in

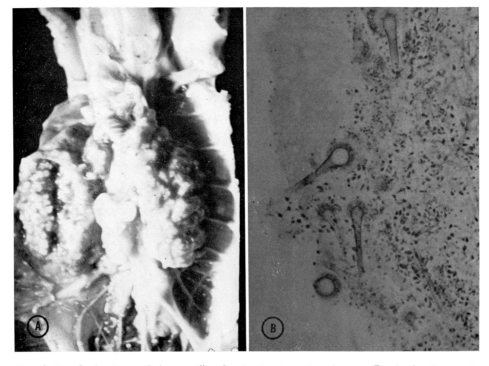

Fig. 6–3. **A.** Lesions of *Aspergillus fumigatus* in avian lungs. **B.** *A. fumigatus* in lung of a grouse.

a flock. Mortality is low. The signs are anorexia, gasping or coughing, and a rapid loss of body weight.

Aspergillosis should be suspected at necropsy if a bright, greenish yellow, caseous exudate is present in the lungs or air sacs. Gross evidence of inflammatory processes are observable in the lungs. The air sacs are thickened. Raised nodules of inflammatory exudate and mycelia are commonly present in the air sacs and in the lungs. They vary in size and number, usually are yellowish to yellowish white and are sometimes described as "button ulcers." The center or the entire mass may be necrotic.

Histologic examination reveals the bronchi, bronchioles and alveoli to be filled with mucus, mycelia, fibrin, and leucocytic and inflammatory cells. Foreign body giant cells may be observed. The parenchyma shows an exudative cellular inflammation where it has been penetrated by mycelia. Hyphae are 4 to 6 μ in diameter, septate, and dichotomously branched. Elements of conidiophores may be found in the air passages but not in the tissues.

Clinical signs which have been described in domestic and pet animals do not differ materially from pneumonia of other causes. Elevated temperature, mucopurulent nasal discharges, conjunctivitis, and coughing or sneezing are more or less constant manifestations.

The pathology of aspergillosis in a calf has been described by Eggert and Romberg.[11] Grossly and histologically, the liver and lymph nodes had no significant

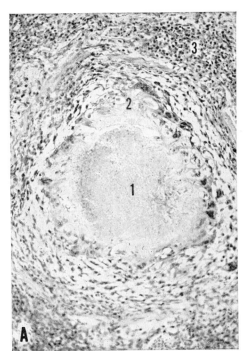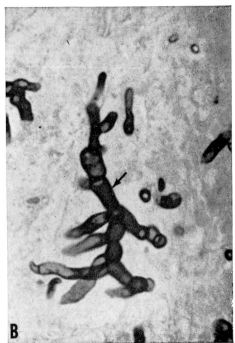

Fig. 6–4. Aspergillosis. **A.** Granuloma in lung of a chick ($\times$ 185). Necrotic center (1) of the granuloma is surrounded by giant cells (2) and lymphocytes (3) in connective tissue. **B.** Gridley fungus stain of a section ($\times$ 840) to demonstrate the septate, branching fungus. AFIP 164237. Contributor: Dr. C. L. Davis (Smith, Jones and Hunt, Veterinary Pathology, courtesy of Lea & Febiger)

changes, but the lungs had multiple discrete granulomas, often with necrotic centers. Microscopically, in the necrotic areas, there were occasional aggregates of polymorphonuclear leukocytes surrounding brightly eosinophilic, radiating, clublike structures which, on casual inspection, resembled the "sulphur" granules of actinomycosis and actinobacillosis. However, hyphae-like structures were seen under higher magnification, both in cross section and sagittally, at the centers of the radiating clubs. Sections stained with Gomori's stain showed numerous branching septate hyphae in the lesions.

Bovine mycotic abortions usually occur from the third through the eighth month of pregnancy. The aborted fetus is rarely alive. Placentae are retained in approximately 60 percent of the cases.

Grossly, the placental lesions of bovine mycotic abortion due to *Aspergillus fumigatus* show yellow to grey cotyledons which are markedly thickened especially in the periphery. In some instances, the intercotyledonary tissue appears leathery and is grey to tan in color. The number of affected cotyledons is variable. Typically, a necrotizing placentitis is observed with the most severe changes in the cotyledons. Extensive necrosis may occur with polymorphonuclear infiltration around the necrotic areas and diffuse distribution throughout the placenta. Edema and hemorrhage are common and extensive. Arteritis is generally present and hyphae may be seen invading the vessel walls.[16]

Some aborted fetuses appear normal on gross examination. Those grossly affected usually show circumscribed, raised, grey lesions which resemble "ringworm." Hillman[16] has described the skin lesions as focal areas of necrosis with neutrophilic infiltration of the epidermis. He observed fungal hyphae in the necrotic tissue, in the hair follicles and in the adjacent connective tissue.

Sautter and coworkers[19] and more recently Pakes and associates[20] have adequately described the pathology of feline pulmonary aspergillosis.

LABORATORY DIAGNOSIS

The diagnosis of aspergillosis requires a cautious approach. The aspergilli are the most common fungus contaminants in the laboratory, and they can be routinely cultured from the skin and upper respiratory tract of healthy animals. Repeated isolation of an *Aspergillus* species from clinical material in the absence of other pathogenic agents is presumptive evidence of aspergillosis. Recovery of the organism from seared or unexposed tissues helps to support a diagnosis. Further evidence is obtained by the demonstration in tissue of mycelium compatible with *Aspergillus* spp. and diagnosis has often been made on this basis. A combination of cultural and histologic evidence is the firmest basis for diagnosis.

Direct Microscopic Examination

Wet preparations may be examined directly. Material for scrapings is readily available from the air passages of affected birds at necropsy. Smears may be Gram-stained. The mycelium is 4 to 6 μ wide, septate, and of fairly uniform diameter. Although it is not possible (unless a conidial head is present) to distinguish this mycelium from that of other hyaline Eumycetes, the presence of large amounts of such mycelium is suggestive of aspergillosis.[29]

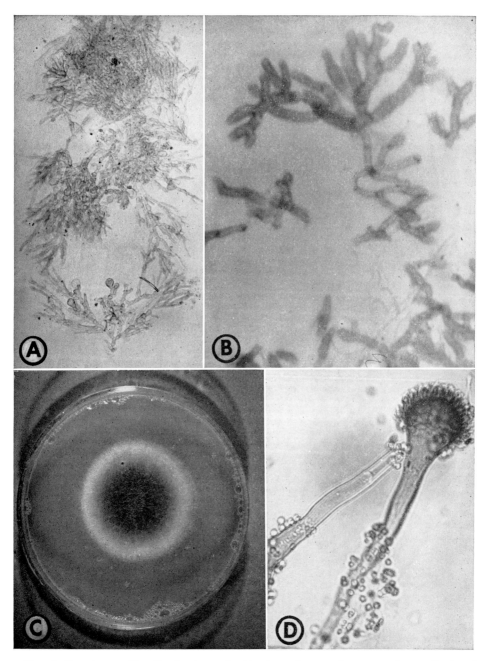

Fig. 6–5. *Aspergillus fumigatus.* **A.** Hyphae from pulmonary tissue digested with NaOH. × 212. **B.** Same as **A.** × 690. **C.** Colony on Sabouraud's agar. **D.** Conidiophore. × 690. (Emmons, Binford and Utz, Medical Mycology, courtesy of Lea & Febiger)

Culture

Aspergillus fumigatus and *A. flavus* as well as other *Aspergillus* spp. grow readily on Sabouraud dextrose agar. Antibacterial antibiotics may be used in the media. Cycloheximide should not be used as most aspergilli are sensitive to this antibiotic.

The colonies of *Aspergillus fumigatus* are rapidly growing and flat. They are at first white and slightly fuzzy, but as the conidia develop they become a dark bluish green and appear powdery. Old cultures have a greyish, "smoky" appearance that is quite characteristic.

On microscopic examination, the vesicle is shaped like an inverted flask with a rounded bottom and a long drawn-out neck. A single row of sterigmata is borne on the upper half of the vesicle in a more-or-less crowded parallel formation. The wall of the conidiophore is smooth when observed under a 100× objective. The conidia are spherical, green and rough-surfaced. The chains of the conidia that arise from the sterigmata are roughly parallel to each other. This gives a columnar or flaglike appearance to the heads.[29]

The colonies of *A. flavus* grow and spread rapidly on ordinary media. Small areas of sterile hyphae may be present in dry areas of the medium. The color of

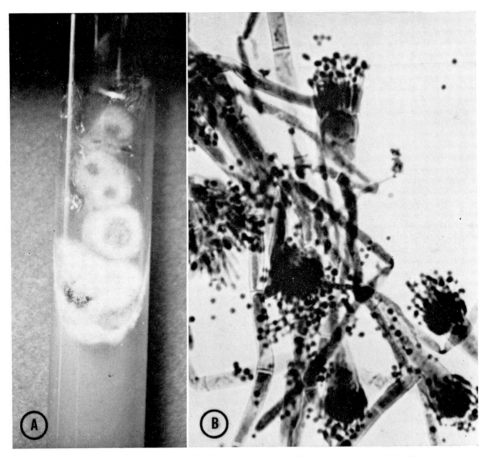

Fig. 6–6. **A.** Young colonies of *A. fumigatus* on Sabouraud agar. **B.** Slide culture of *A. fumigatus,* Cotton Blue stain.

conidial areas varies from light yellowish green to dark green. Green coloration may partially disappear in old cultures with resulting yellow or yellow brown appearance of the surface. The reverse color is yellow, becoming brown with age. Most conidiophores arise from submerged hyphae. They may be 400 to 1000 μ long by 5 to 15 μ in diameter. The conidiophore walls are pitted, rough and sometimes spiny in appearance. They broaden upward and gradually enlarge into vesicles 10 to 30 or 40 μ in diameter, domelike in the smaller heads, flaskshaped in larger heads. Sterigmata are formed either in single series or with both single and double

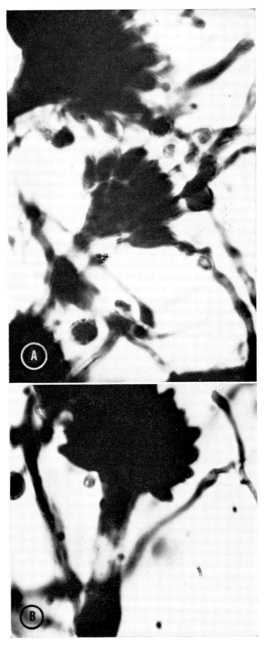

Fig. 6–7. *Aspergillus flavus*. **A.** Note similarity of vesicle and sterigmata to *A. fumigatus.* **B.** High magnification to show rough stalk of *A. flavus,* a feature which aids identification.

series on the same vesicle. The conidia are 3 to 5 μ in diameter, pyriform to round, pitted and echinulated. They vary from nearly colorless to yellowish green.[30]

When other *Aspergillus* spp. are cultured from clinical material, and if there is sufficient basis from direct examination of the clinical materials to suspect that the isolate in question may be the etiologic agent, it is often desirable to make precise identification. Complete descriptions and keys to identification have been prepared in a recent publication by Raper and Fennell.[31]

Pathogenicity Tests

Animal inoculation is not necessary for identification of the agents of aspergillosis.

Immunology

Immunologic tests have not been developed for the diagnosis of aspergillosis in animals. Man is subject to clinical manifestations of sensitivity to antigens of aspergilli. Respiratory symptoms are predominant and are considered to be an allergic response. No analogous condition has been recorded in animals.

Walter and Jones have recently discussed the serologic tests in diagnosis of aspergillosis in man.[35] They compared the complement fixation test with the immunoelectrophoretic test and evaluated skin test antigens.

DIFFERENTIAL DIAGNOSIS

Clinically, aspergillosis of pet and large domestic animals needs differentiation from other mycoses and from respiratory infections of viral etiology. Mycotic bovine abortions may simulate those of brucellosis, vibriosis and leptospirosis.

The disease in birds over two weeks of age may resemble infectious bronchitis, pullorum or the CRD-air sac complex. The acute form of "brooder pneumonia" affects younger chicks and poults. Characteristically, the lungs have numerous granular nodules and the air sacs are thickened and have a greenish, viscous, exudative surface. The lesions are confined to the respiratory system, whereas in pullorum disease, lesions will be present also in the abdominal viscera.

EPIDEMIOLOGY

The aspergilli are worldwide in distribution, and they fulfill an important role in decomposition processes in soil and elsewhere. Their normal life cycle is saprophytic and is not dependent upon parasitism of man or animals for survival. They are prolific spore producers under a wide range of environmental conditions. The airborne dissemination of their spores contributes to their ubiquity and their role as commonly encountered laboratory contaminants. Those species which have been identified as potential pathogens can be recovered easily from air, dust, hay and straw. One wonders that more animals do not become infected, and we can speculate that those which are affected have probably received massive exposure.

In attempts to produce experimental aspergillosis in mice, Sidransky and Friedman[36] observed that the number of animals infected by airborne *Aspergillus flavus* spores could be increased by giving them either antibacterial antibiotics or adrenal cortical steroids, and that the number increased markedly by giving them both. The administration of cortisone and antibiotics or cortisone alone rendered animals highly susceptible to fatal aspergillosis.

The disease is not transmitted from individual to individual or from animals to man.

TREATMENT

No effective treatment exists for avian aspergillosis. Control of the disease requires finding the source of the sporulating fungus—almost invariably in the litter—and as nearly as possible eliminating it. Infection of birds in incubators was formerly a problem, but it has been practically eliminated with modern incubation practices.

REFERENCES

1. Mayer, A. C. and Emmert, G.: Verschimmelung in lebenden Körper. Deutsch. Arch. Anat. Physiol., *1* (1815): 310.
2. Chute, H. L., O'Meara, D. C. and Barden, E. S.: A Bibliography of Avian Mycosis. University of Maine, Misc. Publ. No. 665, 1962.
3. Fiennes, R. N. T.: Penguin Pathology. Int. Zoo Yb., *7* (1967): 11–14.
4. Ainsworth, G. C. and Austwick, P.: *Fungal Diseases of Animals.* Farnham Royal, Bucks, England, Commonwealth Agricultural Bureaux, 1959.
5. Lundvall, R. L. and Romberg, P. F.: Persistent Diarrhea in Colts. J. Amer. Vet. Med. Ass., *137* (1960): 481–483.
6. Mahaffey, L. W. and Adam, N. M.: Abortions Associated with Mycotic Lesions of the Placenta in Mares. J. Amer. Vet. Med. Ass., *144* (1964): 24–32.
7. Meissner, H. and Köser, A.: Das ansteckende Verfohlen und seine Bekämpfung. Deutsche tieraztl. Wchnschr., *41* (1933): 753.
8. Austwick, P. K. C., Gitter, M. and Watkins, C. V.: Pulmonary Aspergillosis in Lambs. Vet. Rec., *72* (1960): 19–21.
9. Gracey, J. F. and Baxter, J. T.: Generalized *Aspergillus fumigatus* Infection in a Lamb. Brit. Vet. J., *117* (1961): 11–14.
10. Davis, C. L. and Schaefer, W. B.: Cutaneous Aspergillosis in a Cow. J. Amer. Vet. Med. Ass., *141* (1962): 1339–1343.
11. Eggert, M. J. and Romberg, P. F.: Pulmonary Aspergillosis in a Calf. J. Amer. Vet. Med. Ass., *137* (1960): 595–596.
12. Griffin, R. M.: Pulmonary Aspergillosis in the Calf. Vet. Rec., *84* (1969): 109–111.
13. Molello, J. A. and Busey, W.: Pulmonary Aspergillosis in a Cow. J. Amer. Vet. Med. Ass., *137* (1963): 632–633.
14. Austwick, P. K. C.: The Presence of *Aspergillus fumigatus* in the Lungs of Dairy Cows. Lab. Invest., *11* (1962): 1065–1072.
15. Bendixen, H. C. and Plum, N.: Schimmelpilze (*Aspergillus fumigatus* und *Absidia ramosa*) als Abortusursache bein Rinde. Acta Path. et Microbiol. Scand., *6* (1929): 252–322.
16. Hillman, R. B.: Bovine Mycotic Placentitis in New York State. Cornell Vet., *59* (1969): 269–288.
17. Hillman, R. B. and McEntee, K.: Experimental Studies on Bovine Mycotic Placentitis. Cornell Vet., *59* (1969): 289–302.
18. Cysewski, S. J. and Pier, A. C.: Mycotic Abortion in Ewes Produced by *Aspergillus fumigatus*. Amer. J. Vet. Res., *29* (1968): 1135–1151.
19. Sautter, J. H., Steele, D. S. and Henry, J. F.: Aspergillosis in a Cat. J. Amer. Vet. Med. Ass., *127* (1955): 518–519.
20. Pakes, S. P., New, A. E. and Benbrook, S. C.: Pulmonary Aspergillosis in a Cat. J. Amer. Vet. Med. Ass., *151* (1967): 950–953.
21. Chute, H. L. and Barden, E.: The Fungous Flora of Chick Hatcheries. Avian Diseases, *8* (1964): 12–19.
22. Stock, B. L.: Case Report: Generalized Granulomatous Lesions in Chickens and Wild Ducks caused by *Aspergillus species*. Avian Diseases, *5* (1961): 89–93.
23. Walker, J.: Aspergillosis in the Ostrich Chick. Union of S. Africa, Dept. Agri. Ann. Rpts., Dir. Vet. Research, *3–4* (1915): 535–574.

24. Durant, A. J. and Tucker, C. M.:   Aspergillosis of Wild Turkeys Reared in Captivity. J. Amer. Vet. Med. Ass., *86* (1935): 781–784.

25. O'Meara, D. C. and Chute, H. L.:   Aspergillosis Experimentally Produced in Hatching Chicks. Avian Diseases, *3* (1959): 404–406.

26. McDiarmid, A.: Aspergillosis in Freeliving Wild Birds. J. Comp. Path. Ther., *65* (1955): 246–248.

27. Rosen, M. N.: Aspergillosis in Wild and Domestic Fowl. Avian Diseases, *8* (1964): 1–6.

28. Eggert, M. J. and Barnhart, J. V.: A Case of Egg-Borne Aspergillosis. J. Amer. Vet. Med. Ass., *122* (1953): 225.

29. Ajello, L., Georg, L. K., Kaplan, W. and Kaufman, L.:   *Laboratory Manual for Medical Mycology*. Washington, U.S. Govt. Printing Office, 1963.

30. Thom, C. and Raper, K. B.:   *A Manual of the Aspergilli*. Baltimore, Williams & Wilkins Company, 1945.

31. Raper, K. B. and Fennell, D. I.:   *The Genus Aspergillus*. Baltimore, Williams & Wilkins Company, 1965.

32. Hewer, T. F., Pearson, H. and Wright, A.:   Aspergillosis and Mucormycosis in Two Newborn Calves of *Okapia johnstoni* (Sclater). Brit. Vet. J., *124* (1968): 282–286.

33. Jasmin, A. M., Carroll, J. M. and Baucom, J. N.: Pulmonary Aspergillosis of the American Alligator (*Alligator mississippiensis*). Amer. J. Vet. Clin. Path., *2* (1968): 93–95.

34. Olson, L. D.: Case Report: Aspergillosis in Japanese Quail. Avian Diseases, *13* (1969): 225–227.

35. Walter, J. E. and Jones, R. D.: Serologic Tests in Diagnosis of Aspergillosis. Dis. Chest, *53* (1968): 729–735.

36. Sidransky, H. and Friedman, L.:   The Effect of Cortisone and Antibiotics on Experimental Pulmonary Aspergillosis. Amer. J. Path., *35* (1959): 169–183.

Part III
THE SYSTEMIC MYCOSES

CHAPTER 7 | Coccidioidomycosis

Coccidioidomycosis, caused by the dimorphic fungus *Coccidioides immitis*, is primarily a respiratory disease of a variety of animals and man. Infections vary through a wide spectrum from an inapparent or benign entity to a progressive, disseminated and fatal form. There is a marked variation in susceptibility among the various animal species; primates and dogs are the most susceptible.

HISTORY, GEOGRAPHIC DISTRIBUTION AND PREVALENCE

Posadas[1] reported the first case of coccidioidomycosis in man from Argentina in 1892. Skin lesions which he thought were neoplastic contained an organism that he likened to the protozoan *Coccidia*. Subsequently he reported upon the production of experimental infections, by inoculation of infected tissue or exudate into monkeys and dogs, and stated that the monkey was particularly susceptible to the disease, dying in 20 to 30 days after inoculation.[2]

The first North American case was described by Rixford from California in 1894 as a protozoic dermatitis.[3] Rixford and Gilchrist[4] recorded the results of animal experimentation in which local lesions and lymphadenitis followed inoculations into the skin of dogs and rabbits. Only localized cutaneous coccidioidal lesions developed in the infected animals. They also attempted bacteriologic culture but discarded their culture plates as contaminated when they became rapidly overgrown with a mold. They believed that the offending organism was a protozoan of the class Sporozoa which they called *Coccidioides immitis* ("im," not; plus "mitis," mild).

Animal inoculation studies reported in 1900 helped Ophuls and Moffit to establish that the "protozoan" of Rixford and Gilchrist was actually a fungus.[5] They also had considered the mold on their culture plates to be a contaminant until subcultures from inoculated guinea pigs regularly showed the same fungus. In a continuing study Ophuls found that intraperitoneal inoculation of the fungus into guinea pigs produced progressive granulomatous lesions in the abdominal viscera and testes while lesions that resulted from subcutaneous inoculation remained localized.[6]

Naturally occurring coccidioidomycosis in animals was first reported in California by Giltner in 1918.[7] He described the fungus in the mediastinal and bronchial

7

lymph nodes of cattle slaughtered at an abattoir. With his bovine fungal isolate, he was able to infect guinea pigs, rabbits, dogs, cattle, sheep and swine and noted a decreasing susceptibility within the various species in about the order named.

In 1929 Beck described coccidioidal lesions in a sheep and six cases in cattle.[8] Two cases in cattle were described by Traum the same year.[9] Beck and associates[10] reported 10 more cases in cattle in 1931. It is noteworthy that all naturally occurring animal cases recorded prior to 1933 had occcurred in California and only mediastinal and lymph node involvement had been observed.

Coccidioidomycosis was diagnosed in a heifer slaughtered at the Denver stockyards in 1931. The case was reported by Stiles and coworkers in 1933.[11] The animal had been shipped from a feedlot in northern Colorado; however, details of its origin were not available. The disease was again diagnosed at Denver in 1935 in a single steer from a group of 35 that were raised in New Mexico and fed in Arizona.[12]

Pulmonary coccidioidal granuloma in cattle was described by Davis, Stiles and McGregor in 1937.[13] This was the first report of granulomatous lesions in bovine lungs. The affected animals also had a history of feedlot exposure in the endemic area. Like all the natural animal cases previously reported, none of the animals showed signs of clinical disease or dissemination of infection beyond the pulmonary lymph nodes.

That the dog is susceptible to experimental coccidioidomycosis was first reported by Posadas[2] in 1900 and subsequently by other early workers.[4,7] The first naturally acquired canine case was described from Tucson, Arizona by Farness in 1940.[14] This was also the first animal case reported in which dissemination had occurred. Multiple nodules were present in the liver, spleen and kidneys in addition to the lungs. In the latter site, some of the nodules were necrotic and spherules believed to contain ascospores were present in the lesions.

Smith[15] described a case of disseminated coccidioidomycosis in a dog which died in Iowa in 1946 after having resided at Eagle Pass, Texas for more than a year. During the residency in Texas, it was twice under the care of a veterinarian for an ailment which was diagnosed as a throat infection and which caused dysphagia and loss of appetite. Spriegel and Milliff[16] diagnosed another canine case from Corpus Christi, Texas which they reported in 1948.

Twenty-five confirmed cases in dogs from the Tucson, Arizona area were reported by Reed in 1954.[17] He cited three additional cases previously reported from California. He also evaluated the intradermal use of coccidioidin, a sterile filtrate prepared from a synthetic broth medium in which several strains of *Coccidioides immitis* had been grown. This skin test antigen was useful in delineating the endemic areas and also was an aid in the diagnosis of canine coccidioidomycosis. In a subsequent report, Reed[18] studied an additional 27 cases provided by cooperating practitioners from the Tucson and Phoenix areas of Arizona. He further evaluated the diagnostic use of coccidioidin skin sensitivity, as well as the use of precipitin and complement fixation tests for detecting humoral antibodies. He also outlined the course, age and breed susceptibility, symptomatology and common necropsy findings as a means of facilitating recognition of the disease in dogs.

Most of the early cases of canine coccidioidomycosis dealt only with the disseminated form of the disease. More recent publications have established that a benign, nonprogressive form occurs also in dogs. Levan and Burger described a case of primary pulmonary coccidioidal disease similar to the "valley fever" (a mild

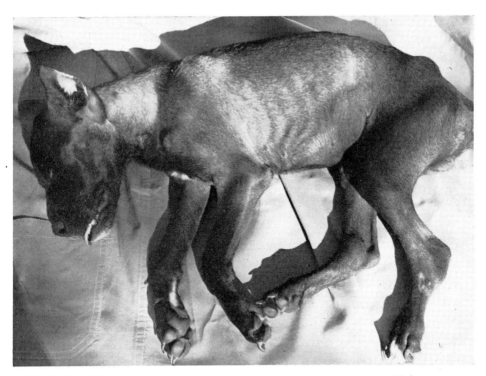

Fig. 7–1. Disseminated coccidioidomycosis in a three-month old boxer pup. Lungs were a mass of scar tissue. Note typical skeletal lesion of left hock. (Courtesy of Dr. R. E. Reed.)

upper respiratory form of coccidioidomycosis common in man in the San Joaquin Valley of California), from which the dog completely recovered.[19] Necropsy studies were conducted on a group of 34 stray dogs selected at random from a dog pound.[20] All were apparently healthy except one which appeared to have distemper. Coccidioidal lesions were found in the lungs and hilar lymph nodes of eight.

An epizootic among five related, purebred collies that had been moved from Detroit, Michigan to the endemic area near Tucson was reported by Ajello and colleagues.[21] The signs and course of the disease seen among members of the group spanned a spectrum as broad as the range of symptoms seen in man. One of the dogs had an acutely fatal infection, one died after an illness of several months' duration, one received euthanasia after a long illness, one initially responded to treatment and, after exacerbation occurred, gradually recovered, and one recovered rapidly after a brief illness.

A study of nonfatal cases by Reed[22] and an extensive study of 100 disseminated cases by Maddy[23] contributed significantly to the understanding of the high prevalence and wide range of forms of canine coccidioidomycosis in endemic areas. They observed that the majority of disseminated cases occurred in dogs less than two years of age and that boxers and Doberman pinschers appeared to be more susceptible to dissemination than other breeds. The similarity of the disease in the dog and man was noted, as was the possibility of using dogs for research.

The high incidence of bovine coccidioidomycosis in certain areas was determined almost concurrently with the discoveries of the prevalence of the disease in dogs. Prchal[24] in 1948 recounted 511 cases found in cattle slaughtered under Federal inspection during a 10-month period in Phoenix. These cases represented 1.3 percent of all cattle processed during the observation period. No lesions were found outside the thoracic cavity and none were of sufficient extent to warrant condemnation of the carcass. Prchal observed that lesions were not seen in animals shipped from pasture and suggested there was strong evidence that the infection was acquired in dusty feedlots. He noted the extreme aridity of the region and compared the geographic conditions in the Salt River Valley of Arizona with the counties of California that Beck had previously mentioned as being endemic.

Maddy[25] made another extensive study which included over 3000 bovine cases observed during the course of meat inspection at various abattoirs in southern California. The infection was found in 1.8 percent of all cattle inspected (calves excluded), in 2.9 percent of all beef steers and heifers and in 7.3 percent of the steers and heifers from San Joaquin Valley feedlots. He confirmed Prchal's observation that the disease was not common in dairy cattle on green pasture. In the same publication he delineated the known areas of endemicity for man and indicated that the disease is enzootic in cattle in approximately the same areas.

In a superb ecologic study, Maddy[26] showed a close correlation between the geographic areas of the Lower Sonoran Life Zone and the known endemic areas for coccidioidomycosis in the United States. His report helped others to find and delimit the geographic areas of endemicity in Mexico and Central and South America.

The presently known general areas of endemicity include much of the San Joaquin Valley and the southern desert counties of California, relatively small areas in the southernmost parts of Nevada and Utah, extensive areas in the southern parts of Arizona and New Mexico, and the southwestern and west-central parts of Texas. A high endemicity is anticipated in the arid regions of northern Mexico, particularly in those states adjacent to the U.S.-Mexico border.

The known areas in South America include the northwestern part of Venezuela and the Gran Chaco Pampa region of Argentina and Paraguay. There is a possibility, based on climatic similarities, that this region extends into southern Bolivia.

In Central America the Comayagua Valley in the central part of Honduras has been known to be endemic for several years, and animal and human cases have recently been described from the Motagua River Valley in Guatemala by Mayorga.[27] He suggests the possibility of the disease existing in Nicaragua by citing the report of coccidioidomycosis being found in a dog in Norway soon after arriving there from Nicaragua. The disease has not been found in autochthonous cases in either Costa Rica or Panama.

Sporadic infections have been reported from other parts of the world but endemicity has not been established and it would appear that the disease was "imported" or that infections resulted from fomite transmission. The known endemic areas have been precisely and meticulously detailed by Fiese[28] in his excellent monograph. He has described the loci of highest endemicity, and a remarkable correlation exists with the incidence of animal cases occurring in those regions.

Infections in animals have been reported only infrequently from countries other than the United States. That the disease occurs with high frequency in animals in other endemic areas appears to be a valid postulation. Also, the probability of other endemic and enzootic areas being discovered seems predictable, for soil and climatic conditions favorable to the fungus exist elsewhere in the world.

The diagnosis of coccidioidomycosis in dogs and cattle occurs so frequently in the southwestern United States that most cases are not now reported. Such is not the case with other animal species in which infections have not often been recognized. Maddy[29] made a comprehensive review of animal cases which, in addition to dogs and cattle, included burros, sheep, a horse, a monkey, a gorilla, a chinchilla and several species of wild rodents. His report covered new cases in cattle, sheep, dogs, a llama, a burro, horses, swine and a tapir. Subsequent to Maddy's report, Straub and associates[30] described coccidioidomycosis in three coyotes trapped near Tucson, Arizona.

Infection of cats with *Coccidioides immitis* was not reported until 1963 when Reed and colleagues[31] described two cases which had been discovered in 1960. The fact that the cases occurred in a highly endemic area where veterinarians are alert to the incidence of the disease in other pets, and that no new cases were discovered in the three years intervening between the diagnoses and the report, would indicate that clinically recognizable coccidioidal infection is quite uncommon in cats.

CLINICAL SIGNS AND PATHOLOGY

It seems quite certain that only a very few of the total number of animals in endemic areas exposed to spores of *Coccidioides immitis* ever show clinical signs. Indeed, several species apparently never show clinical evidence of disease, e.g., cattle, sheep and swine. This does not represent species non-susceptibility, for affected thoracic lymph nodes are frequently found in these animals during routine carcass examination following slaughter. The high degree of resistance of these species is attested by the fact that no cases of disseminated coccidioidomycosis have ever been reported in these animals.

In subhuman primates and dogs, the most susceptible animal species, the disease

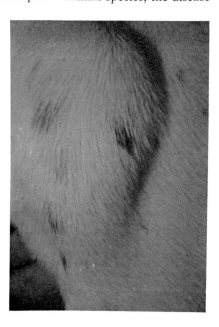

Fig. 7–2. Coccidioidomycosis with superficial node involvement.

is generally a self-limited pulmonary infection, but it may become widely disseminated. Converse and his associates[32] have observed that the dog is as susceptible to the disease as the monkey; the dog, however, is more resistant to its effects by virtue of an ability to maintain a blood supply to the lesions for a longer period of time and because of a faster and more prolific collagen response. The high incidence of infection in dogs is partly attributable to the common habits of tracking and sniffing the ground and digging and investigating the depths of rodent burrows. Other than rodents in which the infection is quite common,[33] dogs live in more intimate contact with the fungus-containing soil than do other domestic and pet animals. With rare exceptions, it is only the dog in which clinically important coccidioidomycosis occurs.

Skin test surveys of normal dogs, with no history of previous respiratory illness, have shown that many become infected without ever exhibiting signs of illness.[29] The great majority of these are thought to attain a durable immunity. Some dogs in which dissemination eventually occurs do not show signs of the primary phase of the infection, others exhibit a wide range of clinical signs. Reed studied the case histories of a number of dogs, presented to clinics in endemic areas, in which the owners had observed listlessness, poor appetite, intermittent diarrhea, cough, shortness of breath, loss of weight, lameness, enlarged joints, atrophy of muscle groups, and exhibition of pain in various parts of the body.[18] Coughing was the most common sign observed, and it varied from strong and harsh to soft and shallow. The coughs were typically dry and unproductive, yielding exudate from the respiratory passages in few cases. The more prominent respiratory signs result from granulomatous enlargement of lymph nodes adjacent to the upper respiratory tract.

If dissemination from the thoracic cavity is going to occur in the dog, it is most likely to become apparent at about four months after infection, but it can follow shortly after the primary illness or not until several years later. With dissemination, sometimes gradual cachexia occurs, and there may be intermittent diarrhea as well

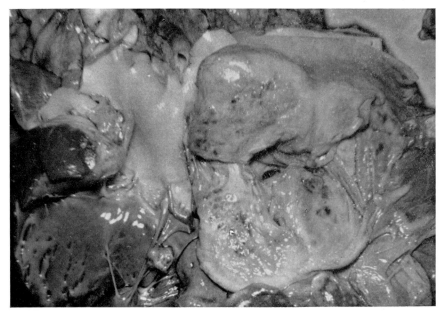

Fig. 7–3. Coccidioidal granulomata in canine mediastinal lymph node.

as various circulatory disturbances. The temperature may follow an erratic elevated course. Bone involvement which occurs frequently, may result in marked lameness and, eventually, painful invalidism. At this point dogs are usually humanely destroyed, but they can live on for several months if given considerable nursing.[29]

At necropsy the gross lesions may be found confined to the lungs or widely disseminated beyond the thoracic cavity. (Exceptions to dissemination have been noted previously for certain species.) The liver, spleen and kidneys are affected often and, in the dog, bones are affected commonly with granulomas developing at the epiphysial junction. Some leg-bone lesions of long duration produce sinuses which drain through the skin. It is noteworthy that the gross and microscopic pathology of coccidioidomycosis is very similar in man and dog, except in regard to bone lesions. In man the lesions tend to be more destructive in type, whereas in the dog they are more proliferative.[23]

The gross lesions of coccidioidomycosis have been described by many writers as resembling those of tuberculosis in many respects. They may appear as discrete or confluent granulomas, with or without suppuration. White to greyish nodules of various size may be found in the lungs, lymph nodes, liver, spleen, meninges, bone marrow and other organs. The nodules are usually irregular in size and shape and may or may not yield an exudate if put under pressure. They often feel firm and dense to the touch, give the impression of connective tissue and are found frequently in close relationship to the large blood vessels.

The causative organism appears in the tissues of its host as a round, doubly-walled structure commonly called the "spherule"; it has a remarkable resemblance to a coccidial oocyst. Most spherules measure in the range from 10 to 80 μ in

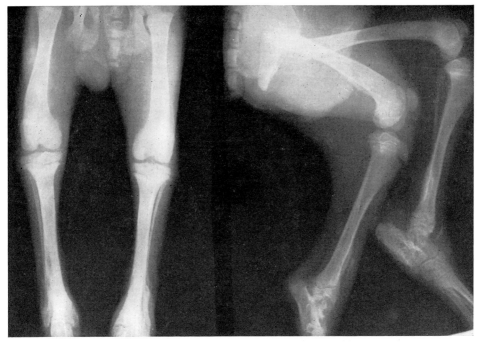

Fig. 7–4.   Osteomyelitis distal right tibia and tibial crest separation.   Canine coccidioidomycosis.   (Courtesy of Dr. R. E. Reed)

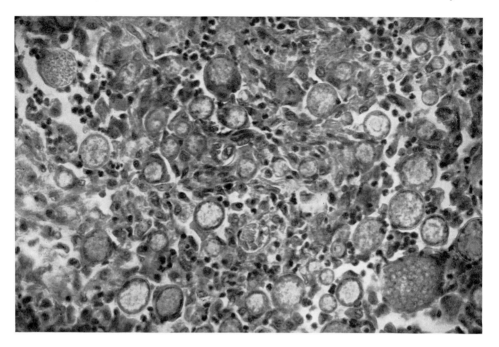

Fig. 7–5.   *Coccidioides immitis* in bone of a dog.   Various stages of sporulation are represented.   (Courtesy of Dr. C. H. Bridges)

diameter with an occasional one attaining a size of 200 μ or more.   Its doubly refractile wall is about 2 μ thick.   When mature, it contains round or irregular endospores, from a few to several hundred, sometimes located peripherally, but more commonly throughout the spherule.   Endospores are usually 2 to 5 μ in diameter, but may occasionally reach 30 to 40 μ.

Endospores are released into the surrounding tissue by "rupture" of the spherule wall, and each endospore gradually enlarges and develops into a new spherule.   The cycle is repeated until the process is arrested by the defense mechanisms of the host.   Because of the manner of multiplication (endosporulation), more young than mature spherules are commonly seen in tissue and these have clear cytoplasm and appear without granules or endospores.   Spherules in all stages of maturation may be present in the tissue and this accounts for the mixed tissue reactions observed.   The newly released endospore elicits an acute inflammatory response in the immediate area with a resulting suppurative reaction in which the tissue becomes rich in neutrophils.   With enlargement of the endospore, the reaction gradually becomes more chronic and lymphocytes replace the neutrophils.   As the spherule continues to develop, macrophages appear in company with plasma cells and large mononuclear cells.   Eventually a more chronic reaction develops where epithelioid cells are the more predominant type.   Mature spherules are usually found in giant cells or histiocytes of the host.

Smith[15] gave the first complete description of the histologic changes in disseminated canine coccidioidomycosis, and the many reports are well-represented by the words he used to describe his case:

Microscopic sections revealed the granulomatous nature of the lesions. The predominant cell was reticulo-endothelial in type, large, usually rather well-rounded, and with a very generous amount of acidophilic cytoplasm. The nuclei were pale and vesicular, often indented, and more or less eccentrically placed. Macrophagic activity was evidenced by the rather frequent occurrence of lymphocytes and polymorphonuclear leukocytes within these cells. Polymorphonuclear neutrophils and lymphocytes also were important elements in the reactive tissue. Very commonly all three types of cells were intimately and rather uniformly intermingled, but in other areas there was a tendency for the polymorphonuclear cells to be gathered together to form tiny purulent foci. There were no giant cells and no necrosis or calcification. Stroma, or connective tissue elements, were minimal and inconspicuous, although small, well-filled blood vessels were rather numerous. Sharp boundaries separated the granulation tissue from the normal structures which it was invading, but encapsulation, as a rule, did not occur. In the lung there were some areas where the new tissue was almost entirely fibrous, but even here it did not encircle the reticulo-endothelial areas.

Only a very few cases of equine coccidioidomycosis have been reported. The first recorded case was described by Zontine,[34] and a study of the pathologic changes in the same horse was later made by Rehkemper.[35] He noted the resemblance of the symptoms and lesions, in this widely disseminated case, to those seen in many dogs with dissemination. A later equine case, reported by Crane,[36] had no gross lesions outside the thorax, with the exception of an ulcerative abscess over the xiphoid cartilage.

Three cases of chronic progressive disseminated equine coccidioidomycosis have been reported from California recently.[43] All were characterized by granulomatous peritonitis and pleuritis, with little involvement in parenchymatous organs. One case was diagnosed ante mortem by culture of *Coccidioides immitis* from thoracic and abdominal fluids.

The clinical signs and pathologic lesions observed in cats do not differ markedly from those of dogs. One of two recorded cases was free of temperature and respiratory distress. The prominence of multinucleated giant cells in the lesions examined microscopically differed from the usual canine case. Both cats had cutaneous lesions, but primary infection through the skin has never been proved in animals.[31]

LABORATORY DIAGNOSIS

A discussion of the procedures for handling *Coccidioides immitis* in the laboratory should be introduced with a warning concerning the dangers of infection to laboratory personnel. Fiese stated that handling the mycelial form of *Coccidioides immitis* without proper precautions is foolhardy and for members of certain races may be suicidal.[28] His reference to racial differences is of special concern to Negroes and Filipinos, for Negroes are more than 10 times and Filipinos more than 150 times as prone to suffer disseminated coccidioidomycosis as are Caucasians.

The hazard lies in the possibility of inhaling spores from the mycelial form (usual culture form) of the fungus. Mature mycelial filaments fragment into tiny arthrospores which readily become airborne following the removal of a cotton plug or the lifting of a petri dish cover. For this reason, the use of petri dishes for culturing the fungus is generally proscribed. Some laboratories immediately autoclave any white fluffy culture suspected of being *Coccidioides immitis*. Others make transfers to liquid media from cultures suspected of being *C. immitis* while the young colonies are still moist, and before the aerial mycelium has developed. The handling of the mold form of the fungus can be eliminated by inoculating suspected clinical material into mice. The resulting infected tissues or exudates, which are less dangerous to handle, can be collected and examined for spherules. Clinical material should be treated with antibacterial antibiotics before it is inoculated, to prevent contaminating bacteria from killing the experimental animal.

The danger of inhalation of arthrospores can be greatly reduced by handling the fungus in a protective hood, preferably in one that exhausts through an incinerator. Some mycologists routinely handle the cultural form for transfer or to obtain material for animal inoculation after wetting down the aerial growth in culture tubes with sterile saline. The saline is introduced through a hypodermic needle carefully inserted between the culture tube and cotton plug.

Cultures for gross demonstration can be killed by inverting them above a solution of formaldehyde in a closed container for 24 hours at 37° C. Formalinized tube cultures are excellent material for students to make slide preparations from for microscopic examination.

Direct Microscopic Examination

Direct, unstained mounts of clinical materials such as urine, exudates, and pleural or peritoneal fluids may contain characteristic spherules. These, when mature, have a thick refractile wall and contain endospores. If the preliminary examination is unrewarding, a drop of exudate may be mixed with a drop of saline, then covered with a coverslip and sealed with vaseline. The preparation is allowed to stand for several hours, and if spherules or endospores are present, sprouting hyphae may be observed emerging from them.

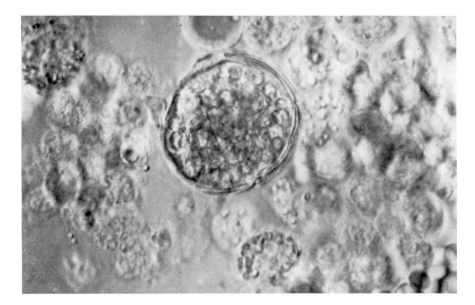

Fig. 7–6. Sporulating spherule of *Coccidioides immitis* in pus from draining sinus in dog's shoulder. (Courtesy of Dr. C. H. Bridges)

Culture

Clinical material should be inoculated onto several slants of selective medium such as cycloheximide-chloramphenicol agar. This medium selectively isolates *Coccidioides immitis* from among almost all other bacteria and saprophytic fungi. All cultures should be in cotton plugged tubes and incubated at room temperature.

Coccidioides grows faster than most pathogenic fungi, and growth is usually evident in three to five days. The colony is at first moist, flat and grey and to a degree resembles the colonies of some bacteria. In the next few days a fluffy white aerial mycelium develops. As the colony matures, it becomes covered with a thick, tangled, cottony mycelium. Some areas of the colony may appear flat with sparse growth. As the colony ages the surface color gradually changes to tan or light brown, and its surface becomes powdery with fragmented hyphae and free arthrospores. Many variations of the typical colony, both grossly and microscopically, have been described.[37]

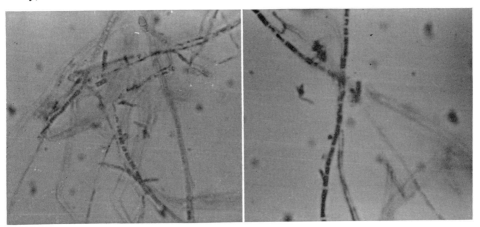

Fig. 7–7.   Arthrospores in *Coccidioides immitis* mycelial hyphae. Cotton Blue stain.

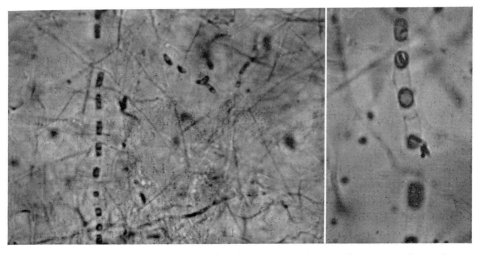

Fig. 7–8.   Arthrospores in old *Coccidioides immitis* cultures. Spores tend to enlarge and often have a lessened uniformity of arrangement in old cultures.

Material for microscopic identification should not be removed from the tube until after it has been flooded to prevent the dispersion of infectious spores into the air. After wetting, a small portion of the mycelial mat is transferred into a drop of lacto-phenol-cotton blue stain previously placed on a glass slide and is then carefully topped with a coverslip. The characteristic arthrospores are seen as thick-walled barrel or cask-shaped enlargements of the hyphae alternately spaced between smaller, empty cells. The spores vary between 2 and 10 μ in diameter and have a tendency to be larger and with a lessened uniformity of arrangement in old cultures. The hyphal chains break up into fragments and individual arthrospores quite readily.

The mycelial form can be converted to the spherule or tissue form *in vitro* using a specialized medium and technic.[38] The procedure is, however, not readily adaptable to diagnostic work.

Pathogenicity Tests

Animal inoculation studies are performed for several purposes: to establish the pathogenicity of a particular isolate, to avoid handling the mycelial form as a safety precaution, to convert the mycelial form to the tissue form and to confirm the tentative identification of a mycelial culture. There are several nonpathogenic soil inhabiting fungi that have a gross resemblance to *Coccidioides immitis*, and some of them produce arthrospores with a confusing resemblance.[39] It is mandatory that suspicious cultures be confirmed by animal inoculation to make a positive identification.

Both mice and male guinea pigs are satisfactory for inoculation. Mice should receive 1.0 ml. of mycelial suspension, or suspended spherule-containing material, by intraperitoneal inoculation; guinea pigs are inoculated with 0.1 ml. intratesticularly. After four to six days, spherules can be demonstrated in pus from the resulting peritonitis or orchitis. Mice will succumb in 10 to 14 days with lesions in the omentum, spleen and lungs. Demonstration of endosporulating spherules by histologic examination confirms the identity of the fungus.

Immunology

Immunologic tests for coccidioidomycosis have been an aid not only in diagnosis but also in helping to establish the geographic limits of endemic areas. The most used technic has been skin testing with coccidioidin. Much of the early survey and evaluation work was accomplished with antigen furnished through the courtesy of the late Dr. Charles E. Smith, University of California, who made monumental contributions to the knowledge of coccidioidomycosis. Coccidioidin is now commercially available.

The test is performed in the animal by intradermal inoculation of 0.1 ml. of undiluted coccidioidin. An area of induration at the inoculation site in excess of 5 mm. in diameter is considered positive. Larger areas of induration and severe reaction with necrosis may occur in dogs. The test is read at 24 to 48 hours in omnivorous and carnivorous animals and at 72 to 96 hours in herbivorous animals. It is believed that immunity to coccidioidomycosis is almost lifelong and skin sensitivity usually persists for many years. The skin test may be negative in some disseminated cases. At the onset of infection an animal may be skin test negative.

A few weeks later, if tested, conversion to a positive skin test constitutes positive diagnosis.[29]

Coccidioidin is used also as the test antigen in those laboratories performing the precipitin and complement fixation (CF) tests. The precipitin test needs refinement and at present is not routinely done in diagnostic laboratories. The reliability of the CF test is limited, since dog serums are frequently anticomplementary. Kaplan has applied the fluorescent antibody technic to the laboratory diagnosis of coccidioidomycosis and recommends it for testing anticomplementary serums.[40]

A latex particle agglutination test and a gel diffusion precipitin test have recently been evaluated as screening tests for the diagnosis of canine coccidioidomycosis.[51]

DIFFERENTIAL DIAGNOSIS

With an increasing awareness of the incidence of systemic mycoses, particularly in dogs, these diseases are being considered more frequently in diagnosis. Those animals with persistent coughs or with other respiratory ailments that fail to respond to therapy should be suspected of having pulmonary fungus disease. Gradual progression to cachexia with diarrhea that is intermittent, persistent, or which responds only temporarily to medication is justification for giving consideration to disseminated mycotic infection. Coccidioidomycosis may be confused with histoplasmosis and blastomycosis; primary infections need differentiation from respiratory infections of viral etiology.

Thoracic radiographs may be a valuable diagnostic aid. Properly exposed film will reveal the abnormal processes associated with thoracic coccidioidal infection, principally widening (sunburst) hilar shadows, increased density along the bronchial tree, and nodular lesions in the lung parenchyma. This picture has come to be considered pathognomonic of the disease in dogs from the enzootic areas.[18]

EPIDEMIOLOGY

The work of Maddy,[26] previously referred to, graphically describes the climatic conditions necessary for the survival and propagation of *Coccidioides immitis* in the soil. He stated that apparently the fungus can grow only where there is a definite period of very hot weather when there is little or no rainfall. During this time the surface soil becomes somewhat sterilized. *C. immitis* seemingly remains viable just below the sterile layer of soil, as well as in the moister and more nitrogen-rich environment of desert rodent holes. When rain eventually falls, the humidity in the surface soil probably approaches the optimum for the growth of the fungus. *C. immitis* then grows well until other soil microorganisms interfere with its growth or until the soil dries. The fungus probably still grows for a while down in cracks and holes until the humidity in these sites drops and/or other soil microorganisms interfere with its growth. Then the environment is the most infective with winds picking up dust and arthrospores and carrying them about. A study of prevailing winds over the entire endemic area does not give any overall clue to the spread of this fungus. Possibly the fungus cannot remain viable for long periods of time when airborne. A majority of human and animal infections seem to occur during the windy, dusty weather following the wet season. The sun again begins sterilizing the surface soil and the infection rates begin to drop. Infections can still occur in the seasons between peaks of infectivity. These are sometimes associated with soil digging and the subsequent exposure to viable spores. Infections are often seen in dogs that dig in rodent holes while hunting on the desert, or that are taken into new home subdivisions where the soil has been graded.

Coccidioidomycosis is acquired by both man and the lower animals as the result of the inhalation of the infected dust prevalent in endemic areas. Infection can also result from inhalation of spores following fomite transport and with unequivocal certainty from careless handling of cultures of the mold form. The disease is not transmitted from individual to individual or from animals to man.

One report of animal-to-animal transmission under unusual circumstances has been described.[42] An infant monkey was found to have a primary pulmonary infection apparently after inhaling exudative material from a draining sinus on its mother's forearm. The mother had previously been experimentally infected at the site of the sinus.

TREATMENT

To date there is no chemotherapeutic agent available that consistently gives satisfactory results in the treatment of deep mycotic infections of animals. Amphotericin B has been rather extensively used, but it may cause severe undesirable side effects. In some cases it apparently is more harmful than beneficial. Dogs receiving an experimental dose of 1.0 mg./kg. daily, administered intravenously, developed a high incidence of emesis, hematemesis and anorexia. Those surviving medication showed additional signs of toxicity in the form of an increased blood urea nitrogen (BUN) and a decrease in phenolsulfonphthalein excretion by the kidney and bromsulphalein excretion by the liver.[44]

Cats are more intolerant of amphotericin B than are dogs. A single intravenous injection may elicit both renal and pulmonary dysfunction. To the authors' knowledge, successful use of this drug in cats has never been reported. In this species, its use has invariably been disappointing at the Texas A. & M. Clinic, and one of the clinicians has stated that in cats, amphotericin B is a synonym for euthanasia.[45]

Many of the animals treated at this clinic have been presented as referrals. On admission, several have been dehydrated and cachectic. This has biased our evaluation of amphotericin B therapy. However, it points out the need for early diagnosis and careful supervision of the patient during therapy. Anorexia, weight loss and dehydration are consistently problems associated with long term amphotericin B therapy in dogs. However, the major problem is nephrotoxicity, and this should be continuously monitored. The duration of therapy has to be weighed against potential kidney damage. This is an encouragement to shorten therapy time. Some dogs which have been discharged as apparently "cured" have had severe exacerbations after weeks or months and have been readmitted as terminal cases.

The side effects of amphotericin B therapy often may be reduced to a tolerable level by administering small aliquots initially and gradually increasing to a maintenance therapeutic level. Also, dogs often tolerate 1.0 mg./kg. of the drug every other day better than 0.5 mg./kg. given daily. For these reasons, it is recommended that 0.05 mg./kg. be given in the initial dose. The injections are continued every other day or three times weekly and each dose is increased by 0.05 mg./kg. until the fifth injection when 0.25 mg./kg. is given. The 0.25 mg. dosage is maintained three times weekly depending upon the response, kidney function and general condition of the patient. A BUN determination should be obtained at least once, and preferably twice weekly. Therapy should be temporarily discontinued if the BUN rises above 75.0 mg./100 ml. The daily dose may be diluted to a volume of 5 ml. in 5-percent dextrose in saline and should be given intravenously. It has previously been recommended that a minimum of 100 ml. of diluent and very slow administration be used to alleviate renal intoxication.[46] The restraint necessary, time and hazard of using large volumes seem to outweigh the possible advantages.

Reed has recommended an evaluation of progress when the cumulative dose of amphotericin B reaches 5.0 mg./lb. and cautious use of extended medication. The problem of renal damage must constantly be weighed against benefits of treatment.

Butler and Hill[47] have successfully given dogs larger doses than those recommended above over extended periods of time. Apparently normal dogs were the subjects of their studies. Reed has administered larger doses to experimentally infected dogs starting on the day of infection.[48]

As previously stated, the cautious therapy regimen recommended by the writer is biased by results obtained in dogs with advanced systemic mycoses. Probably those with less debility and those with pulmonary involvement only would tolerate more intensive medication.

Because of the renal toxicity of amphotericin B, perhaps clinicians should consider the use of stilbamidine or other aromatic diamines in the treatment of blastomycosis. Recently Lockwood and associates[49] reported on 10 years' experience in the treatment of North American blastomycosis in man, and they stated that stilbamidine isethionate continues to be a useful therapeutic agent.

Apparently there are no reports of the successful use of amphotericin B in bovine cryptococcal mastitis. Its use seems warranted in valuable animals. A colleague has reported limited success with intramammary infusions of an aqueous solution of 1:5000 acriflavine. Pounden and coworkers used and evaluated various sulfonamides and antibiotics.[50] They obtained best results with generally recommended methods for the control of mastitis, including segregation of infected animals, improved sanitation and limited treatments, coupled with care in milking machine operation and some changes in feeding practices.

REFERENCES

1. Posadas, A.: Ensayo anatomopatologico sobre una neoplasia considerada como micosis fungoidea. An. Circ. Med. Argent., *15* (1892): 8.
2. Posadas, A.: Psorospermose Infectante Generalise. Rev. Chir., Paris, *21* (1900): 277–282.
3. Rixford, E.: A Case of Protozoic Dermatitis. Occidental M. Times., *8* (1894): 704–707.
4. Rixford, E. and Gilchrist, T. C.: Two Cases of Protozoan (Coccidioidal) Infection of the Skin and Other Organs. Johns Hopkins Hosp. Rep., *1* (1896): 209–268.
5. Ophuls, W. and Moffitt, H. C.: A New Pathogenic Mould (formerly described as a protozoon: *Coccidioides immitis* pyogenes): Preliminary Report. Philadelphia M. J., *5*, (1900): 1471–1472.
6. Ophuls, W.: Further Observations on a Pathogenic Mould Formerly Described as a Protozoon (*Coccidioides immitis*, Coccidioides pyogenes); J. Exp. Med., *6* (1905): 443–486.
7. Giltner, L. T.: Occurrence of Coccidioidal Granuloma (Oidiomycosis) in Cattle. J. Agri. Res., *14* (1918): 533–542.
8. Beck, M. D.: Occurrence of *Coccidioides immitis* in Lesions of Slaughtered Animals. Proc. Soc. Exp. Biol. Med., *26* (1929): 534–536.
9. Traum, J.: Coccidioidal Granuloma. J. Amer. Vet. Med. Ass., *28* (1929): 478–479.

10. Beck, D. M., Traum, J., and Harrington, E. S.: Coccidioidal Granuloma: Occurrence in Animals—Reference to Skin Tests. J. Amer. Vet. Med. Ass., *31* (1931): 490–499.
11. Stiles, G. W., Shahan, M. S. and Davis, C. L.: Coccidioidal Granuloma in Cattle in Colorado. J. Amer. Vet. Med. Ass., *35* (1933): 928–930.
12. Stiles, G. W. and Davis, C. L.: A Case of Bovine Coccidioidal Granuloma from the Southwest. J. Amer. Vet. Med. Ass., *40* (1935): 582–585.
13. Davis, C. L., Stiles, G. W., and McGregor, A. N.: Pulmonary Coccidioidal Granuloma; A New Site of Infection in Cattle. J. Amer. Vet. Med. Ass., *44* (1937): 209–215.
14. Farness, O. J.: Coccidioidal Infection in a Dog. J. Amer. Vet. Med. Ass., *97* (1940): 263–264.
15. Smith, H. A.: Coccidioidomycosis in Animals, with Report of a New Case in a Dog. Amer. J. Path., *24* (1948): 223–233.
16. Spriegel, J. M. and Milliff, J. H.: Coccidioidomycosis in a Dog. J. Amer. Vet. Med. Ass., *112* (1948): 244.
17. Reed, R. E.: Serology and Coccidioidin Skin Testing in Diagnosis of Canine Coccidioidomycosis. Proc. Book. A.V.M.A., 91st Ann. Meet., Seattle (Aug. 23–26, 1954): 199–203.
18. Reed, R. E.: Diagnosis of Disseminated Canine Coccidioidomycosis. J. Amer. Vet. Med. Ass., *128* (1956): 196–201.
19. Levan, N. E. and Burger, C. H.: Coccidioidomycosis in Dogs; A Report of Three Cases. Calif. Med., *83* (1955): 379–380.
20. Straub, M. and Schwarz, J.: Coccidioidomycotic Thoracic Lesions in Dogs in Tucson, Arizona. Arch. Path., *62* (1956): 479–488.
21. Ajello, L., Reed, R. E., Maddy, K. T., Burdurin, A. A. and Moore, J. C.: Ecological and Epizootiological Studies on Canine Coccidioidomycosis. J. Amer. Vet. Med. Ass., *124* (1956): 485–490.
22. Reed, R. E.: Nonfatal Coccidioidomycosis of Dogs. Proc. Sympos. Coccid., U.S. Pub. Health Serv., Pub. No. 575 (1957): 101–104.
23. Maddy, K. T.: A Study of One Hundred Cases of Disseminated Coccidioidomycosis in the Dog. Proc. Sympos. Coccid., U.S. Pub. Health Serv., Pub. No. 575 (1957): 107–118.
24. Prchal, C. J.: Coccidioidomycosis of Cattle in Arizona. J. Amer. Vet. Med. Ass., *112* (1948): 461–465.
25. Maddy, K. T.: Coccidioidomycosis of Cattle in the Southwestern United States. J. Amer. Vet. Med. Ass., *124* (1954): 456–464.
26. Maddy, K. T.: Ecological Factors Possibly Relating to the Geographic Distribution of *Coccidioides immitis*. Proc. Sympos. Coccid., U.S. Pub. Health Serv., Pub. No. 575, (1957): 144–157.
27. Mayorga, R.: Coccidioidomycosis in Central America. Proc. of 2nd Coccid. Sympos., University of Arizona Press (1965): 287–291.
28. Fiese, M. J.: Coccidioidomycosis. Springfield, Charles C Thomas, Publisher, 1958.
29. Maddy, K. T.: Coccidioidomycosis in Animals. Vet. Med., *54* (1959): 233–242.
30. Straub, M., Trautman, R. J. and Greene, J. W.: Coccidioidomycosis in 3 Coyotes. Amer. J. Vet. Res., *22* (1961): 811–813.
31. Reed, R. E., Hoge, R. S. and Trautman, R. J.: Coccidioidomycosis in Two Cats. J. Amer. Vet. Med. Ass., *143* (1963): 953–956.
32. Converse, J. L., Reed, R. E., Kuller, H. W., Trautman, R. J., Snyder, E. M., and Ray, J. G.: Experimental Epidemiology of Coccidioidomycosis: I. Epizootiology of Naturally Exposed Monkeys and Dogs. Proc. of 2nd Coccid. Sympos., University of Arizona Press (1965): 397–402.
33. Emmons, C. W.: Coccidioidomycosis in Wild Rodents; A Method of Determining the Extent of Endemic Areas. Public Health Rep., *58* (1943): 1–5.
34. Zontine, W. J.: Coccidioidomycosis in the Horse—A Case Report. J. Amer. Vet. Med. Ass., *132* (1958): 490–492.
35. Rehkemper, J A.: Coccidioidomycosis in the Horse. A Pathologic Study. Cornell Vet., *49* (1959): 198–211.
36. Crane, C. S.: Equine Coccidioidomycosis. Case Report. Vet. Med. *57* (1962): 1073–1074.

37. Huppert, M., Sun, S. H., and Bailey, J. W.: Natural Variability in Coccidioides Immitis. Proc. of 2nd Coccid. Sympos., University of Arizona Press (1965): 397–402.
38. Converse, J. L.: Effect of Physico-chemical Environment on Spherulation of Coccidioides Immitis in a Chemically Defined Medium. J. Bact., *72* (1956): 784–792.
39. Emmons, C. W.: Fungi Which Resemble Coccidioides Immitis. Proc. of 2nd Coccid. Sympos., University of Arizona Press (1965): 333–337.
40. Kaplan, W.: Application of the Fluorescent Antibody Technique to the Diagnosis and Study of Coccidioidomycosis. Proc. of 2nd Coccid. Sympos., University of Arizona Press (1965): 227–231.
41. Elconin, A. F., Egeberg, M. C., Bald, J. G., Matkin, A. O. and Egeberg, R. O.: A Fungicide Effective Against Coccidioides Immitis in the Soil. Proc. of 2nd Coccid. Sympos., University of Arizona Press (1965): 319–321.
42. Castleberry, M. W., Converse, J. L. and Del Favero, J. E.: Coccidioidomycosis Transmission to Infant Monkey from Its Mother. Arch. Path., *75* (1963): 459–461.
43. DeMartini, J. C. and Riddle, W. E.: Disseminated Coccidioidomycosis in Two Horses and a Pony. J. Amer. Vet. Med. Ass., *155* (1969): 149–156.
44. Hildick-Smith, G., Blank, H., and Sarkany, I.: *Fungus Diseases and Their Treatment.* London, J. & A. Churchill Ltd., 1964.
45. Gowing, G. M.: Associate Professor of Veterinary Medicine & Surgery, Texas A. & M. University, College Station, Texas.
46. Jungerman, P.: Diagnosis and Treatment of Animal Mycoses. Southwest. Vet., *18* (1965): 101–103.
47. Butler, W. T. and Hill, G. J.: Intravenous Administration of Amphotericin B in the Dog. J. Amer. Vet. Med. Ass., *144* (1964): 399–402
48. Reed, R. E.: "Coccidioidomycosis," in *Current Veterinary Therapy III, Small Animal Practice* (Kirk, R. W., Ed.). Philadelphia, W. B. Saunders Company, 1968.
49. Lockwood, W. R., Allison, F., Jr., Blair, E. B., and Busey, J. F.: The Treatment of North American Blastomycosis—Ten Years Experience. Amer. Rev. Resp. Dis., *100* (1969): 314–320.
50. Pounden, W. D., Anderson, J. M., and Jaeger, R. F.: A Severe Mastitis Problem Associated with *Cryptococcus Neoformans* in a Large Dairy Herd. Amer. J. Vet. Res., *13* (1952): 121–128.
51. Yturraspe, D. J.: Clinical Evaluation of a Latex Particle Agglutination Test and a Gel Diffusion Precipitin Test in the Diagnosis of Canine Coccidioidomycosis. J. Amer. Vet. Med. Ass., *158* (1971): 1249–1256.

CHAPTER 8 | Histoplasmosis

Histoplasmosis, caused by the dimorphic fungus *Histoplasma capsulatum*, is primarily a pulmonary and occasionally a fatal disseminated disease in man and animals. The etiologic agent grows intracellularly as a yeast which has an affinity for the reticuloendothelial cells of its host. In nature and at temperatures below 35° C. it grows in a mycelial form. The dog is the most susceptible of the lower animals; clinically apparent and disseminated infection is rare in animals other than the dog.

HISTORY, GEOGRAPHIC DISTRIBUTION AND PREVALENCE

Dr. S. T. Darling[1] discovered the causative agent of histoplasmosis in Panama and described it in 1906. He was searching for an American form of Leishmania and assumed that the intracellular organisms which he saw were protozoan. He noted however, that no kinetoplast was visible and believed he was seeing a new organism which he named *Histoplasma capsulata* (now *capsulatum*). The intracellular organisms he saw in *"histio"*-cytes resembled *"plasmo"*-dium and seemed to have a *capsule*.

Histoplasmosis was first recognized in the United States by Riley and Watson[2] who described a case from Minnesota in 1926. Their report was the first well-documented evidence that the disease was not confined to the tropics. The true fungus nature of *Histoplasma capsulatum* was unknown to the early investigators; however, that it had a greater similarity to a yeast than a protozoan was suggested by da Rocha-Lima[3] in 1912. He also pointed out that Darling's description of flagellate forms of *H. capsulatum* was probably in error.

A total of only six human cases, all in adults and all found post mortem, had been reported prior to diagnosis of the disease in a living infant by Dodd and Tompkins in 1932. In the description of their case which was published in 1934,[4] they gave credit for diagnostic assistance to Dr. Henry E. Meleney[5] who had an unusual interest in both visceral leishmaniasis and histoplasmosis. Dr. Dodd's patient was hospitalized at the Vanderbilt University School of Medicine where Dr. William A. DeMonbreun held an appointment in the Department of Pathology. He was advised of the diagnosis and was prepared upon demise of the infant to make cultures for the organism on a variety of bacteriologic and mycologic media.

106

DeMonbreun's report[6] in 1934 must be classed as a masterpiece. He successfully cultured the fungus from splenic tissue obtained at autopsy and proved its dimorphism by growing it in both its yeast (parasitic) and mycelial (saprophytic) forms. He proved his isolate to be the etiologic agent of histoplasmosis by animal inoculation studies in which he infected monkeys, puppies and mice with the yeast form. He fulfilled Koch's postulates in these experiments. He converted the yeast form to the mycelial form and discovered that only the latter form would grow over a wide temperature range on unenriched media. He was able to convert the mycelial form to the yeast form by passage through animals (monkeys and mice). He described the cultural morphology and nutritional requirements of the organism so completely that he left little work in those areas to be done. In his discussion he stated, "Judging from its cultural characteristics, the saprophytic form of *Histoplasma capsulatum* probably exists free in nature."

An unsuccessful attempt was made by DeMonbreun to change the name of the disease to cytomycosis. He contended that Darling had implied a protozoan parasite as the etiologic agent when he named the disease histoplasmosis. After ascertaining the fungus etiology, he proposed the name cytomycosis of Darling as a substitute. He stated that the new name emphasized the outstanding characteristic of the disease, namely, that there is a generalized infection of the reticuoendothelial system with the occurrence and probable proliferation of the parasitic form of the fungus within these cells. Meleney was a strong proponent for the proposed name change,[7] but it did not attain general acceptance.

DeMonbreun also contributed significantly to the veterinary aspect of lhistoplasmosis in 1939 when he diagnosed the first naturally occurring case of the disease in a dog and proved it by culture.[8] A tentative diagnosis had been made on a biopsy specimen from the liver obtained before death. Confirmation was established by culturing the fungus from antemortem blood and from tissues obtained at necropsy. He discussed the probability that the disease was more common than was generally suspected, and he suggested the possibility that the disease might occur in an unrecognized relatively mild or nonfatal form.

The second authentic case of canine histoplasmosis was reported from St. Louis, Missouri by Callahan[9] in 1944. The diagnosis was based on the presence of the organism associated with histopathologic changes in the spleen and mesenteric lymph nodes.

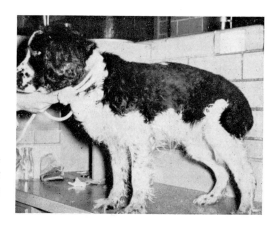

Fig. 8–1. Generalized canine histoplasmosis. Lymphadenopathy and spreading of posterior ribs were prominent signs.

Birge and Riser[10] described two cases from Iowa in 1945; in the same year Tomlinson and Grocott[11] discovered the disease in a dog in the Canal Zone, in the same laboratory and hospital where Darling's original human case was found. It is of interest that the Canal Zone report gave an early clue to some epidemiologic knowledge concerning bat guano. Some weeks before death, the dog had been observed eating dirt around flower bushes that had been fertilized with "bat droppings."

Canine histoplasmosis was diagnosed in 1946 in Brazil by Para[12] and in Virginia by Seibold[13] and by Olson and colleagues.[14] Only ten cases were diagnosed in the eight years following DeMonbreun's original report, but this limited number of reports began to establish the endemic areas for animal histoplasmosis in the Americas.

Natural infection with *Histoplasma capsulatum* was known to occur only in man and dogs until Emmons and associates[15] cultured the organism from rats and a mouse in 1947. The mouse was trapped at a location in Virginia where a dog with histoplasmosis had lived. No gross lesions were observed in the rodents from which *H. capsulatum* was isolated.

Three published cases of naturally occurring canine histoplasmosis were recorded from Missouri during 1948.[16,17] Menges[18] cited four additional cases from Missouri, Michigan and Tennessee. This latter group included the second case diagnosed by DeMonbreun. Reports of histoplasmosis in dogs appeared with increasing frequency after 1948. Menges summarized the descriptions of the disease in an additional 25 cases discovered in the ensuing three years, and the states of Kansas, Indiana and Ohio were added to the expanding area where proved canine cases were diagnosed.[18] A review of histoplasmosis in 1963 mentioned 481 canine cases.[19] Almost all had been found in the central and eastern-central part of the United States; one case each had occurred in Brazil, the Panama Canal Zone and Venezuela.

Cases of histoplasmosis in animals other than the dog have been infrequently reported in the literature, and accounts of disseminated infection are quite rare. In 1950 in Hawaii Adler[20] first discovered bovine histoplasmosis in lung tissue from a range bull that had been submitted to his laboratory by a meat inspector. The entire carcass had been condemned under suspicion of tuberculosis. The diagnosis was based on histopathologic study of the affected tissue. It is assumed that the bull was not obviously sick and had passed antemortem inspection. A second case was reported from Missouri in 1951.[21] The subject was an aged cow that was sick for several months prior to showing terminal signs of dyspnea, diarrhea, swelling of the brisket and grinding of the teeth. Evidence of a concurrent traumatic reticulitis—that may have predisposed the dissemination of the fungus—was observed at necropsy. A decade later *Histoplasma capsulatum* was isolated from bronchial lymph node tissue of a five-month-old calf[22] which had died suddenly with lesions suggestive of blackleg or a similar clostridial infection. Cultures of lung tissue, which had been obtained during a comprehensive survey of animal tissues in Kentucky, were negative for the fungus.

Equine histoplasmosis was first reported in a colt by Richman[23] from Tennessee in 1948. The animal had a history of a respiratory illness that had responded to sulfonamide therapy approximately one month prior to death. No attempt was made to culture the fungus. In 1951, Randall and co-workers[24] discovered yeast cells apparently morphologically identical to *Histoplasma capsulatum* in equine cell cultures. They were cultivating horse spleen and amnio-allantoic membrane by the coverglass method and had obtained their explant tissues from an apparently healthy, adult horse. Three additional equine cases were discovered during the previously mentioned survey of animals in Kentucky. All were diagnosed following necropsy. One was an experimental animal and the others had gross evidence of other disease.

Epizootic lymphangitis of horses, caused by the dimorphic fungus *Histoplasma* (or *Zymonema, Cryptococcus, Saccharomyces, Blastomyces*) *farciminosum*, poses a diagnostic problem in certain parts of the world because its tissue (yeast) form is indistinguishable from that of *H. capsulatum*. Da Rocha-Lima[3] first observed the similarity of the parasitic yeast cells of *H. farciminosum* and *H. capsulatum*. The disease is sometimes called pseudoglanders and the infection is endemic in Equidae in Asia and the countries bordering the Mediterranean.

Ordinarily lesions are confined to the skin, subcutaneous tissues and lymph vessels and nodes. The disease is usually chronic and affected animals become debilitated and cannot be worked. Spontaneous recovery sometimes occurs and complete immunity results.[25]

Although several cases have been reported in the United States, none have been proved by culture and there is doubt concerning their validity;[26] Hagan believed that most of these, possibly all, were cases of sporotrichosis which it resembles clinically.[27]

Emmons described the first isolation of *Histoplasma capsulatum* from a cat in 1949.[28] The animal was one of a group of 49 collected over a two-year-period in Loudoun County, Virginia. Four others in the group were proved positive by culture. The fungus was isolated from the spleen in only one animal; in the other four the isolation was from one or more of the cervical lymph nodes. The author

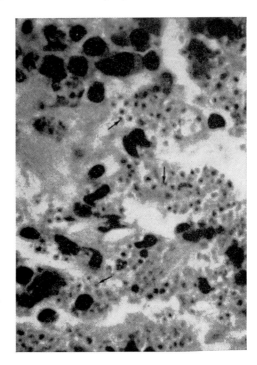

Fig. 8–2. Epizootic lymphangitis, skin of a mule (× 1200). Large numbers of *Histoplasma farciminosum* (arrows) are seen in macrophages. AFIP 134820. Contributor: Ninth Medical Service Detachment Laboratory, U.S. Army. (Smith, Jones and Hunt, Veterinary Pathology, courtesy of Lea & Febiger.)

stated that a surprising feature of histoplasmosis in the cat is the limited extent of the lesions. This observation has been consistent in other studies of cats in endemic areas.[19,29,30] The literature contains only one description of disseminated histoplasmosis in a cat in which clinical signs suggestive of the disease were observed prior to euthanasia of the animal for necropsy.[31]

Clinically evident histoplasmosis has apparently never been described in sheep. No isolations from this species have ever been reported although one study using fluorescent antibody technics indicated infection, and another study using a skin test antigen showed high sensitivity rates in Missouri sheep.[19] The disease in swine is apparently quite rare also. Skin tests with histoplasmin have shown a very low incidence of infection. Only one isolation has been made from swine. Bronchial lymph node tissue of a young pig that had been housed temporarily in a chicken house was positive for *Histoplasma capsulatum* by indirect culture (mouse inoculation).[22]

Histoplasma capsulatum has been isolated with some frequency from a variety of rodents and wild animals. Clinical evidence of disease in these animals is lacking, and it is probable that they harbor only benign, inapparent infections.[15,19]

Perhaps no disease has attained as complete an understanding in as short a time following identification of its etiologic agent as has histoplasmosis. It was first thought to be a rare tropical infection and then equally rare without tropical limitations; knowledge of its occurrence in large numbers of people and animals has evolved rapidly following DeMonbreun's original work. For a while the disease was thought to be largely confined to the river valleys of the Mississippi and its tributaries. This vast area together with smaller loci in the eastern-central United States are recognized for their high endemicity, but the disease is now known to occur over much of the world. Autochthonous cases of histoplasmosis in man from many parts of the world and skin testing, together with soil studies, have established a global distribution; only China remains as a major region where valid cases of histoplasmosis have not been recorded.[32]

Emmons first reported the occurrence of *Histoplasma capsulatum* in the soil after a two-year search in which he collected 387 samples from farm premises where infected animals had been discovered.[33] After proof of its saprophytic existence in soil, other studies revealed its occurrence as a freeliving agent in soil in many parts of the world.[34]

Skin testing in humans for histoplasmosis was first recorded by Van Pernis and colleagues[35] in 1941. They prepared a broth culture filtrate of a strain of *Histoplasma capsulatum* which had been isolated from laryngeal lesions in a human patient. The filter-sterilized test antigen was injected intradermally into the same patient and into experimentally infected mice. Undiluted material elicited immediate reactions and various dilutions produced positive reactions of the delayed type. No reactions were obtained in control mice and noninfected humans. Other workers, in the same year, proposed that the test antigen be called histoplasmin.[36] Skin testing studies were then conducted in many human and animal groups.[37,38] These, together with animal tissue and soil studies, have enabled workers to identify the almost continuously expanding areas of its known occurrence. The skin test studies especially have helped to identify those areas of high prevalence, and those for both animals and man are, for the most part, where the earliest discovered cases were found.

CLINICAL SIGNS AND PATHOLOGY

Clinically evident histoplasmosis develops in only a very few of the total number of infected animals. Other than the dog, most, if not all, species are infected subclinically only. The benign, inapparent form of the disease may be the only form that occurs in wild animals, rodents and most species of domestic animals. Signs of natural infection have never been observed in sheep. The rare cases of disseminated infection that have been reported in cattle, horses and swine have almost invariably been associated with other diseases. Experimental histoplasmosis has been described in horses, cows, sheep and hogs in which the organisms were given by intratracheal inoculation. All developed positive skin tests and circulating antibodies, but clinical signs were limited to fever and coughing in some of the animals and, at necropsy, gross lesions were observed in the lungs of only one sheep and one horse.[39] The results of experimental inoculation of *Histoplasma capsulatum* into 15 rhesus monkeys were recorded in the same report. Severe disease followed intratracheal and intravenous inoculation; mild infection followed intranasal and no clinical signs of disease followed intragastric administration of the organisms. Two of the monkeys died of disseminated disease. Cats, with extremely rare exceptions, have only subclinical, inapparent infections. Although in one study *H. capsulatum* was isolated from tissues (usually peribronchial lymph nodes) of 81 of 449 cats, they were apparently healthy animals.[30]

Large numbers of dogs with no visible signs of illness have also been proved by culture to be infected with *Histoplasma capsulatum*. Positive skin tests on even larger numbers devoid of history of clinical signs seem to prove that a very high percentage of cases remains subclinical and asymptomatic. On this basis one can postulate that many dogs with "colds" or low grade respiratory distress may have mild histoplasmosis.

The term "disseminated" implies that a primary form of the infection has had precedence. This is probably true, at least in the vast majority of cases, but it has not been proved absolutely. Nevertheless, animals with one or several organs affected outside the limits of the thorax are generally considered to have disseminated infection even though the primary infection, probably in the lungs, was asymptomatic or unrecognized.

Four outstanding clinical signs are used to describe canine histoplasmosis: chronic cough, gradual weight loss, persistent or intermittent diarrhea and irregular

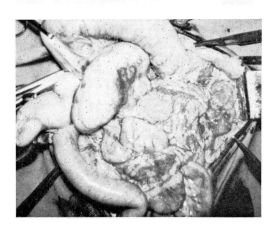

Fig. 8–3. Greatly enlarged mesenteric lymph nodes and thickened intestinal wall in dog with histoplasmosis.

pyrexia. Ascites is a common manifestation with spreading of the posterior ribs and distention of the anterior abdomen. Varying degrees of anemia and icterus are frequently evident. Most of the signs increase in severity as the disease progresses. Lymphadenopathy is commonly detectable and may be the only prominent sign. Splenomegaly and hepatomegaly may occur in advanced cases; less frequently, ulceration of the nasal and oral mucosa occurs. Some dogs will suddenly develop the severe signs of the illness several months following a chronic cough which may have had periods of remission.

At necropsy, gross changes are usually evident. Increased quantities of peritoneal fluid, either turbid or blood-tinged, are often present. The spleen may be enlarged to several times its normal size and be light grey and firm to the touch. The mesenteric lymph nodes are greatly enlarged and sometimes coalesced and appear as a neoplastic mass. Various degrees of enlargement of the liver will be seen. It also is grey and firm. Occasionally light yellow, mottled areas are conspicuous. Gross changes in the genitourinary organs are vague or absent. The adrenals may be enlarged, but usually without gross evidence of focal changes. This is not consistent with histoplasmosis in man where extensive involvement of the adrenal seems to be common. The intestine is often involved and has a thickened wall and a thick nodular, mucosal surface.

The gross postmortem changes seen in the lungs vary from a few discrete nodules in the benign case to extensive nodule formation and occasional cavitation in the severe form. Early focal lesions may appear as hemorrhages. The large nodules are firm and yellowish-white and have been described as having the appearance of metastatic neoplasms.[40] The solitary pulmonary nodule or "histoplasmona," commonly seen in man, is uncommon in dogs; it is situated just beneath the pleura and radiographically resembles a coin-shaped lesion. In dogs, the lymph nodes are usually enlarged, sometimes tremendously. They are firm and uniform in appearance and have been described by Smith and Jones[41] as resembling malignant lymphoma.

Grossly detectable bone involvement apparently never occurs, although invasion of the bone marrow is an almost constant finding in disseminated infections.

Microscopic examination of animal tissues parasitized by *Histoplasma capsulatum* reveals that the organism is found largely intracellularly, particularly in reticulo-endothelial cells (macrophages, endothelioid and epithelioid cells). The fungus grows and reproduces as a yeast in the cellular cytoplasm. The organism is round

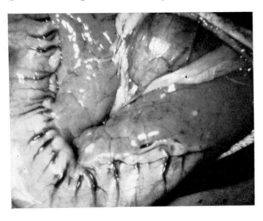

Fig. 8–4. Granulomata in pancreas.
Canine histoplasmosis.

or slightly oval and measures from 1 to 4 μ in diameter. In sections stained with hematoxylin and eosin, a central, spherical, usually basophilic body is surrounded by an unstained zone which, in turn, is encircled by a thin cell wall. This may give the effect of a capsule around the central body, but the organism has no true capsule; the clear halo is actually an artifact due to contraction of the cytoplasm from the wall. By the periodic acid-Schiff (PAS), Bauer's or Gridley's fungus methods, the wall is stained selectively, usually leaving its cytoplasm unstained; thus the organism appears as an empty red ring. These stains are particularly useful in visualizing organisms when only a few are present and in differentiating them from other phagocytized particles, especially tissue debris.[41] The cytoplasm may contain so many organisms that the phagocytizing cell is greatly enlarged. Proliferation of the parasitized cells causes displacement of normal tissues and eventual impairment of physiologic function.

Histopathologic examination of lung tissue and respiratory lymph nodes may reveal encapsulation and healing in dogs with benign infections. The histoplasmic primary focus in dogs (and in man) is often characterized as an acinous, or at most, a lobular pneumonia with subsequent caseation, calcification and encapsulation.[42] The lesions consist of calcified necrotic tissue floating in amorphous chalky material in which many cholesterol clefts may be recognized. Fibrotic capsules containing lymphocytes and mononuclear or epithelioid cells enclose the area and may be hyaline in appearance. The general structure of the lymph node lesions resembles those of the lungs.

In disseminated histoplasmosis, a tendency for the lesions to wall off and encapsulate is lacking. There is, instead, a diffuse cellular reaction with an absence of purulent inflammation and necrosis. The predominant cell is mononuclear with greatly enlarged cytoplasm which often is filled with the characteristic yeast cells.

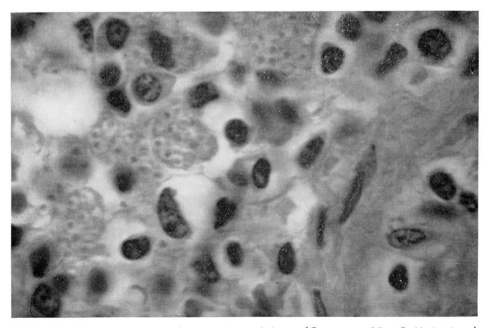

Fig. 8–5. *Histoplasma capsulatum* in lung of dog. (Courtesy of Dr. C. H. Bridges)

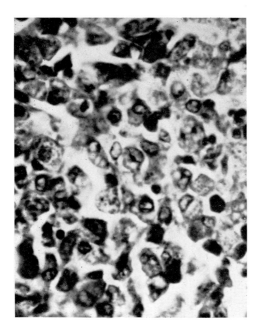

Fig. 8–6. *Histoplasma capsulatum*
in liver of dog.

Plasma cells and lymphocytes are present in smaller numbers throughout the reactive tissue. These accumulations are often in close association with the blood vessels. The lesions may fill the alveoli of the lungs, fill and obstruct the sinusoids of the liver and spleen, or replace the parenchyma. Whatever the tissue or organ involved, the reaction is essentially the same.

LABORATORY DIAGNOSIS

Usually it is not an easy task to isolate *Histoplasma capsulatum* from animal specimens. Sputum, which often yields positive cultures from man, is simply not available from dogs. Gastric washings are difficult to obtain and require heavy tranquilization or anesthesia. All too often only throat swabs or blood samples are submitted to the laboratory for culture. Bacterial contamination complicates isolation of the fungus from the swabs, and the blood contains organisms only in acute disseminated cases.

The number of isolations from dogs could be materially increased if several different types of specimens were cultured. Satisfactory samples of tracheal exudates can be obtained with Tiegland culture tubes. Blood, urine, peritoneal fluid and sternal bone marrow should be requested. Biopsy specimens from affected lymph nodes are useful both for culture and for mouse inoculation. Fecal material should be routinely cultured. Dogs almost invariably swallow the products of their coughing and thus more or less continuously seed the G.I. tract. Also, in disseminated cases, the intestine is often invaded.

All specimens for culture should be freshly obtained. If there is to be a delay before media can be inoculated, the clinical materials should be refrigerated, as the yeast form of *Histoplasma capsulatum* does not remain viable in clinical materials for many hours unless refrigerated or frozen. Whenever possible dry ice should be used for the shipment of clinical materials. Some laboratories accept only media which have been inoculated prior to mailing, unless the clinical materials are shipped in a frozen state.

Direct Microscopic Examination

The examination of unstained clinical material is unrewarding due to the small size and difficulty of differentiation of the organism. Giemsa's or Wright's stains of nodal smears or blood and bone marrow smears in acute disseminated cases may delineate the invading agent.

Culture

For isolation of *Histoplasma capsulatum*, clinical material should be inoculated onto brain heart infusion-cycloheximide-chloramphenicol (BHI-CC) agar and BHI-CC agar fortified with six-percent blood. Incubate both at room temperature and watch for the appearance of white fluffy colonies. Transfer these, if morphologically suggestive of *H. capsulatum*, to screw-capped tubes of BHI and BHI blood agar for 37° C. incubation to confirm by obtaining the yeast form. Do not use media containing cycloheximide and chloramphenicol for incubation at 37° C. These antibiotics, at this temperature, inhibit the yeast forms of the dimorphic fungi.

Inoculation of mice is often helpful in isolating *Histoplasma capsulatum* from clinical material. Fluids, or tissues ground with saline, should be treated with 10,000 units penicillin and 1000 units streptomycin per ml. of material. Incubate at 37° C. for one hour. One ml. of the treated material is inoculated intraperitoneally into two or more mice. These are sacrificed at the end of four weeks and the liver and spleen is cultured on suitable media at room temperature and at 37° C.

Although the use of enriched media is necessary for isolation purposes, since the highly fastidious yeast form of *Histoplasma capsulatum* occurs in clinical materials, the mycelial or saprophytic form of the fungus grows on most culture media at 25–30° C. (room temperature). Sabouraud's media is commonly used and is quite satisfactory for study of the mycelial form of *H. capsulatum*, but some isolates lose the ability to sporulate if continuously transferred on it.

Growth is relatively slow; most isolates require from 10 to 14 days for development of characteristic colonies. The aerial mycelium is at first white and fluffy and it will, in time, cover the surface of the slant. Within a few weeks most cultures change first to a buff and then a brown color. This color change is usually associated with sporulation.

Microscopically, the mycelial structure is generally from 1 to 5 μ in diameter, septate and branched. Both microconidia and macroconidia are formed with a marked variation between strains in the number of spores produced. The smaller microconidia usually appear first. They are round to pyriform, from 2 to 6 μ in diameter, and may be either smooth or echinulated (spiny). The smooth forms usually predominate.

The larger macroconidia (10–25 μ in diameter) are also spherical to pyriform and are characteristically thick-walled and covered with fingerlike or spiny prominences (tubercles) varying from 1 to 8 μ in length. It is these characteristic tuberculate macroconidia, sometimes referred to as "chlamydospores," that serve to identify *Histoplasma capsulatum*. In the first complete description of the fungus, the striking resemblance of the tuberculated spores to the ancient Teutonic war clubs was noted.[6] Some strains fail to produce the characteristic macroconidia. Also, nonpathogenic

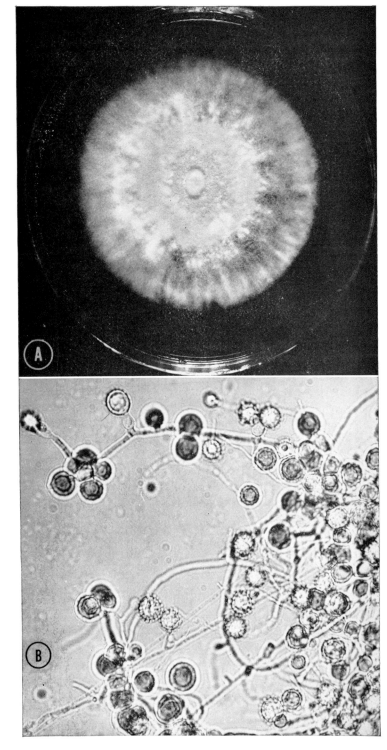

Fig. 8–7. *Histoplasma capsulatum.* **A.** Culture on modified Sabouraud's agar after incubation one month at 30 ° C. **B.** Macroconidia from hyphal form. ✕ 400. (Emmons, Binford and Utz, Medical Mycology, courtesy of Lea & Febiger.)

simulants of the genus *Sepedonium* produce tuberculated spores morphologically similar to those of *H. capsulatum*. This nonpathogenic organism is excellent for classroom study.

Histoplasma farciminosum is a very slowly growing fungus, and it tends to have much less aerial hyphae. The colony is usually grey, moist and has a glabrous (skin-like) surface. When grown on Sabouraud's agar, it produces comparatively short, irregularly curved and branched aerial hyphae and bears only small, irregular, round to oval bodies that are described as "rudimentary aleuriospores." On blood agar, *H. farciminosum* grows on the surface of the medium as a thin, flat, grey, moist colony consisting of relatively few, short, thick segments that possess terminal chlamydospores. In old cultures the chlamydospores frequently become detached from the mycelia to appear as free, thick-walled, spherical structures. These cultural characteristics of *H. farciminosum*, when compared to those of *H. capsulatum*, serve adequately to differentiate the two fungi.[6]

The yeast form (parasitic or tissue form) of *Histoplasma capsulatum* is obtained on enriched media at 37° C. as previously described. The growth range of the yeast form is rather narrow, and at temperatures below 34° C. the yeast generally converts to the mycelial form.

The yeast form cells of young cultures are oval bodies approximately the same size as those seen in tissues (1 to 4 μ). In actively growing cultures, one pole of the cell is pointed; buds may be found at either pole and in some cases bud formation is apolar. As many as three buds may be formed simultaneously from a single mother cell. The cells usually appear round or oval but elongated forms, swollen forms and dumbbell-shaped cells are not unusual. In cultures which are a week or more old, large swollen forms may be observed which are from two to three times the size of actively growing forms and which possess a thick wall and one or more large internal globules of fat.[43]

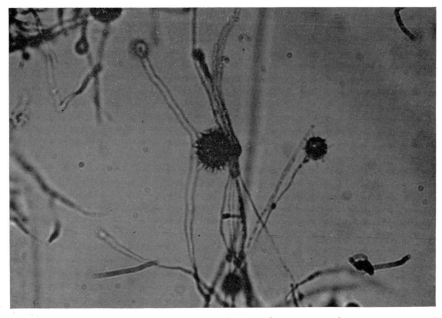

Fig. 8–8.   Slide culture of *Histoplasma capsulatum*.

Conversion of the yeast form to the mycelial form is usually not difficult and can ordinarily be accomplished merely by lowering the incubation temperature. The reciprocal conversion requires an enriched medium (BHI or blood agar), an incubation temperature of 37° C. and adequate moisture. Several transfers of young growth may be necessary to obtain complete conversion. *Histoplasma capsulatum* is a strict aerobe and, if screw-cap tubes are used, they must be periodically loosened. If drying of the slant surface is a problem, sterile nutrient broth or chicken chorioallantoic fluid may be added.

Pathogenicity Tests

Although *H. capsulatum* is pathogenic for a variety of laboratory animals, such tests are not necessary for a positive identification. Culture of the organism in both its characteristic mycelial and yeast forms is conclusive, particularly if conversion of the culture forms is accomplished. DeMonbreun successfully infected puppies, monkeys and mice with his original culture isolate.[6] Many other species have been infected experimentally including guinea pigs, rats, hamsters, gerbils and rabbits. Spontaneous recovery from experimental histoplasmosis has been observed often.[44] The mouse is almost ideal as an experimental animal and has been used to facilitate isolations from tissues, from soil and from heavily contaminated clinical material, and to convert the mycelial form of the fungus to its parasitic form.

Immunology

Although histoplasmosis was originally thought to be invariably a fatal disease in both animals and man, it is now firmly established that the great majority of infected individuals recover with a high degree of immunity. The immunity in dogs may be better even than that in man in which the very young and very old are less resistant. Dogs have a short puppyhood and reach maturity and immunologic competence in a matter of months. For various reasons only a small percentage reach advanced age. These factors may also be involved with other animal species in which fatal histoplasmosis is seen only rarely.

Skin testing of animals with histoplasmin needs critical evaluation. The authors receive many inquiries from veterinarians who question the results of their tests. In many cases they have depended upon the test for a diagnosis. It should be emphasized first that the test is a diagnostic aid only. Recovered animals may react positively. Those in the acute or terminal phases of the disease may be skin-test-negative. The possibility of false positives caused by infection with other mycotic disease agents should also be considered.

Various injection sites have been used for skin testing animals. Sensitivity of the caudal fold and neck areas of cattle have been compared, and the cervical area proved most sensitive. The flank-fold and the medial aspect of the thigh have been injected in dogs, but the cervical test appears to be most satisfactory. Histoplasmin,* diluted 1:100, is injected intradermally after the site is clipped and swabbed with alcohol. One-tenth ml. is injected with a tuberculin syringe and 25–27 gauge needle.

The test is read at 48 hours by observing and palpating the induration or thickening. The induration is measured in the horizontal diameter using a millimeter

* Parke, Davis & Company, Detroit, Michigan.

(metric) scale. A reaction is called positive when there is a definite induration 5 mm. or more in diameter.[38]

Serologic tests for histoplasmosis may be more useful in obtaining a diagnosis than are skin tests. However, the possibility of previous skin tests having produced circulating antibodies should be considered. Histoplasmin and whole yeast-form *Histoplasma capsulatum* cells are two antigens commonly used in complement-fixation (CF) tests for histoplasmosis. Both antigens, though useful, demonstrate cross-reactivity with serums from patients having blastomycosis and coccidioidomycosis.[45] The serologic tests have many of the same limitations as skin tests for supporting a diagnosis, and multiple serum samples obtained from four to six weeks apart are required.

The precipitin test, using histoplasmin as the test antigen, has been used in several serologic studies. The test is not routinely used in diagnostic laboratories. A high precipitin titer can sometimes be demonstrated early in an infection in the absence of CF antibodies or before they appear.

A histoplasmin-latex agglutination test currently has the interest of students and practitioners. The antigen is commercially available and although cross reactions with coccidioidomycosis and blastomycosis occur, it is claimed that they are not as common as in other serologic tests.

DIFFERENTIAL DIAGNOSIS

Histoplasmosis, because of the initial invasion of pulmonary tissue and the proliferative potential of its etiologic agent, mimics many respiratory diseases. Other mycotic diseases should be considered. Canine distemper, nematode (*Filaroides osleri*) invasion of the trachea, kennel cough and canine rickettsiosis merit differential consideration.

In histopathologic sections, the yeast forms of the agents of histoplasmosis and epizootic lymphangitis appear to be identical. Beginning students in pathology have unusual difficulty in differentiating between microscopic lesions of histoplasmosis and toxoplasmosis. Those that succeed develop the ability to recognize the proliferative tissue changes that characterize histoplasmosis; the tissue reaction in toxoplasmosis is essentially necrotizing after rupture of the pseudocysts. Some veterinary pathologists consider the symmetric arrangement of *Histoplasma capsulatum* in infected cells as opposed to a more random arrangement of *Toxoplasma gondii*. A more precise differentiation can be obtained with special fungus stains (PAS, Gridley's or Gomori's methenamine-silver); *Toxoplasma* is not stained by these methods, neither is *Leishmania* which is now being recognized in dogs in the United States. Correction of an erroneous early reference to histoplasmosis in a cat that had toxoplasmosis is credited to Meleney.[46]

African Histoplasmosis

Characteristic cases of infection in man with *Histoplasma capsulatum* have been reported from Africa; a variant which produces "large yeast forms" in tissues has been reported also on that continent by Vanbreuseghem.[47] He named the variant *Histoplasma duboisii*. The mycelial forms of both agents of African histoplasmosis are identical. There are, however, marked differences in the morphology of the tissue or yeast forms of *H. capsulatum* and *H. duboisii*, as well as a difference in the tissue reactions produced. In *H. duboisii* infections, the yeast cells are found pre-

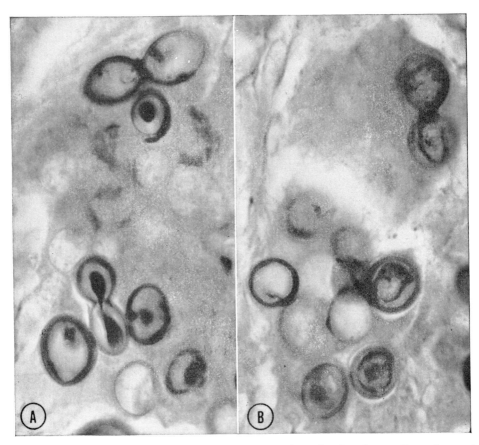

Fig. 8-9. *Histoplasma duboisii*, method of multiplication. Experimental infection in lymph node of hamster. Observe the "hour-glass" cell in the process of nuclear division and the "double" cells not yet separated. **A.** Gridley fungus stain. × 1250. (59-5884). **B.** PAS stain. × 1250. (59-5883). (Emmons, Binford and Utz, Medical Mycology, courtesy of Lea & Febiger.)

dominantly in giant cells, which may reach the size of 80 μ and thus resemble foreign-body giant cells, and the budding cells themselves are extremely large resembling those of *Blastomyces dermatitidis* in size and shape. They vary from 7 to 15 μ in diameter and have thick cell walls from 1.0 to 1.5 μ in thickness.[48]

EPIDEMIOLOGY

DeMonbreun, after proving the existence of a mycelial form of *Histoplasma capsulatum*, stated, "Judging from its cultural characteristics, the saprophytic form of *Histoplasma capsulatum* probably exists free in nature."[6] It was several years before his hypothesis was finally proved, and it required a diligent search before Emmons isolated the fungus from soil in close proximity to a chicken house.[33] Soil isolations became more frequent after other workers detected an association of the fungus with avian habitats.[49] Chickens are apparently not victims of *H. cap-*

sulatum as efforts to infect them experimentally have failed, due presumably to their high normal body temperature. Apparently an enrichment of the soil by chickens' or other birds' fecal droppings gives *H. capsulatum* a competitive advantage over other soil microorganisms. Soils from the roosts of starlings, pigeons and grackles and from caves inhabited by oil birds have yielded many isolations of the organism. The puzzling questions regarding the occurrence of histoplasmosis in urban populations were, to a great extent, answered when these other avian species were found to be involved.

Many species of bats from different parts of the world are also victims of *Histoplasma capsulatum*, and the guano-laden dirt associated with their roosting sites is especially conducive to the growth of the fungus. Isolations have been made from bat tissues and fecal contents.[50] Some bat colonies exist close to human and animal dwellings. Colonies of several thousand may frequent tile roofs, attics, air spaces between inner and outer walls, hollow trees and caves.

In a recent ecologic study, Ajello pointed out that the presence or absence of bat and bird dung in the environment does not solely govern the occurrence and distribution of *Histoplasma capsulatum* in nature. Other ecologic factors must also be at play, for *H. capsulatum* is not invariably present in avian and chiropteran habitats. Throughout the world there are many areas populated with bats and birds that are free from *H. capsulatum*, as determined by negative soil findings and low or negligible levels of histoplasmin reactivity in the population.[32]

Ajello also discussed the temperature ranges, the physical and chemical analyses of the soil and the types of clay minerals present in the soil where *Histoplasma capsulatum* is found. None of the theories he discussed satisfactorily accounts for the indisputable association of *H. capsulatum* with bat and bird habitats and its pattern of geographic distribution. The factors involved must be complex, and much work remains to be done to identify them and to understand their interrelated functions.

Histoplasmosis is acquired by both animals and man from inhalation of the spores of the mycelial form of *Histoplasma capsulatum*. Primary cutaneous infection in man is a rarity,[51] and presumably this is also true in animals. From a practical, clinical viewpoint of animal histoplasmosis, the disease is important only in the dog. Many of the canine breeds are "sniffers and trackers" by nature and are thus prone to massive exposures of the spores. This accounts also for the finding of multiple, primary pulmonary foci in many of the affected dogs.

There is no evidence of transmission of histoplasmosis between individuals or from animals to man. The author is familiar with some veterinary clinics that refuse hospitalization to dogs with suspected systemic mycoses because of a fear that other animals or employees will become infected. Some dogs have been given euthanasia because the owner's fear of contagion has not been alleviated. These practices are unwarranted and need correction.

Soils from which *Histoplasma capsulatum* has been isolated and buildings contaminated with bat and bird feces have been disinfected with three-percent formalin by spraying and soaking.[52] Recommendation of this procedure to pet owners and adoption of its use in animal hospitals should help to mitigate some erroneous conceptions regarding the spread of histoplasmosis.

TREATMENT

See Chapter 7, treatment of systemic mycoses, pp. 102–103.

9

REFERENCES

1. Darling, S. T.: Protozoon General Infection Producing Pseudotubercles in Lungs and Focal Necrosis in Liver, Spleen and Lymph Nodes. JAMA, *46* (1906): 1283–1285.
2. Riley, W. A. and Watson, C. N.: Histoplasmosis of Darling with Report of a Case Originating in Minnesota. Amer. J. Trop. Med., *6* (1926): 271–282.
3. da Rocha-Lima, H.: Histoplasmosis and Epizootische Lymphangitis. Arch. Schiffs. u. Tropenhyg., *16* (1912): 79–85.
4. Dodd, K. and Tompkins, E. H.: A Case of Histoplasmosis of Darling in an Infant. Amer. J. Trop. Med., *14* (1934): 127–137.
5. Meleney, H. E.: The Histopathology of Kala-azar in the Hamster, Monkey and Man. Amer. J. Path., *1* (1925): 147–168.
6. DeMonbreun, W. A.: The Cultivation and Cultural Characteristics of Darling's Histoplasma Capsulatum. Amer. J. Trop. Med., *14* (1934): 93–125.
7. Meleney, H. E.: Histoplasmosis (reticulo-endothelial cytomycosis): A Review with Mention of 13 Unpublished Cases. Amer. J. Trop. Med., *20* (1940): 603–616.
8. DeMonbreun, W. A.: The Dog as a Natural Host for *Histoplasma capsulatum*. Amer. J. Trop. Med., *19* (1939): 565–587.
9. Callahan, W. P.: Spontaneous Histoplasmosis Occurring in a Dog. Amer. J. Trop. Med., *24* (1944): 363–365.
10. Birge, R. F. and Riser, W. H.: Canine Histoplasmosis. Report of Two Cases. No. Amer. Vet., *26* (1945): 281–287.
11. Tomlinson, W. J. and Grocott, R. G.: Canine Histoplasmosis. A Pathologic Study of the Three Reported Cases and the First Case Found in the Canal Zone. Amer. J. Clin. Path., *15* (1945): 501–507.
12. Para, M.: Histoplasmosis in Brazil. Amer. J. Trop. Med., *26* (1946): 273–292.
13. Seibold, H. R.: A Case of Histoplasmosis in a Dog. J. Amer. Vet. Med. Ass., *109* (1946): 209–211.
14. Olson, B. J., Bell, J. A., and Emmons, C. W.: Studies on Histoplasmosis in a Rural Community. Amer. J. Public Health, *37* (1947): 441–449.
15. Emmons, C. W., Bell, J. A., and Olson, B. J.: Naturally Occurring Histoplasmosis in *Mus musculus* and *Rattus norvegicus*. Public Health Rep., *62* (1947): 1642–1646.
16. Harmon, K. S.: Histoplasmosis in Dogs. A Report of Two Cases. J. Amer. Vet. Med. Ass., *113* (1948): 60–62.
17. Anthony, C. H.: Case History—Histoplasmosis Suspect (Canine). Jen-Sal J. (Nov.-Dec. 1948): 22.
18. Menges, R. W.: Canine Histoplasmosis. J. Amer. Vet. Med. Ass., *119* (1951): 411–415.
19. Menges, R. W., Habermann, R. T., Selby, L. A., Ellis, H. R., Behlow, R. F., and Smith, C. D.: A Review and Recent Findings on Histoplasmosis in Animals. Vet. Med., *58* (1963): 331–338.
20. Adler, H. E.: Generalized Infection with a Yeast-Like Fungus in a Range Bull. No. Amer. Vet., *31* (1950): 457–458.
21. Menges, R. W. and Kintner, L. D.: Bovine Histoplasmosis: Case Report. No. Amer. Vet., *32* (1951): 692–695.
22. Menges, R. W., Habermann, R. T., Selby, L. A., and Behlow, R. F.: *Histoplasma capsulatum* Isolated from a Calf and a Pig. Vet. Med., *57* (1962): 1067–1070.
23. Richman, H.: Histoplasmosis in a Colt. No. Amer. Vet., *29* (1948) : 710.
24. Randall, C. C., Orr, M. F., and Schell, F. G.: Detection by Tissue Culture of an Organism Resembling *Histoplasma capsulatum* in an Apparently Healthy Horse. Proc. Soc. Exp. Biol. Med., *78* (1951): 447–450.
25. Blood, D. C. and Henderson, J. A.: *Veterinary Medicine*. 2nd edition, Baltimore, Williams & Wilkins Company, 1963.
26. Saunders, L. Z.: Systemic Fungous Infections in Animals: A Review. Cornell Vet., *38* (1948): 213–238.
27. Bruner, D. W. and Gillespie, J. H.: *Hagan's Infectious Diseases of Domestic Animals*. 5th edition, Ithaca, Cornell University Press, 1966.
28. Emmons, C. W.: Histoplasmosis in Animals. Trans. N.Y. Acad. Sci., Ser. II, *2* (1949): 248–254.

29. Rowley, D. A., Habermann, R. T., and Emmons, C. W.: Histoplasmosis: Pathologic Studies of Fifty Cats and Fifty Dogs from Loudoun County, Virginia. J. Infect. Dis., *95* (1954): 98–108.

30. Emmons, C. W., Rowley, D. A., Olson, B. J., Mattern, C. F. T., Bell, J. A., Powell, E., and Marcey, E. A.: Histoplasmosis: Proved Occurrence of Inapparent Infection in Dogs, Cats and Other Animals. Amer. J. Hyg., *61* (1955): 40–44.

31. Menges, R. W., Furcolow, M. L. and Habermann, R. T.: An Outbreak of Histoplasmosis Involving Animals and Man. Amer. J. Vet. Res., *15* (1954): 520–524.

32. Ajello, L.: Comparative Ecology of Respiratory Mycotic Disease Agents. Bact. Rev., *31* (1967): 6–24.

33. Emmons, C. W.: Isolation of *Histoplasma capsulatum* from Soil. Public Health Rep. *64* (1949): 892–896.

34. Ajello, L.: Geographic Distribution of Histoplasma Capsulatum. In *Histoplasmosis* (Sweaney, H. C., Ed.). Springfield, Charles C Thomas, Publisher, 1960.

35. Van Pernis, P. A., Benson, M. E., and Holinger, P. H.: Specific Cutaneous Reactions with Histoplasmosis. JAMA, *117* (1941): 436–437.

36. Zarafonetis, C. J. D. and Lindberg, R. B.: Histoplasmosis of Darling. Observations on the Antigenic Properties of the Causative Agent. A Preliminary Report. Univ. Hosp. Bull. (Ann Arbor), *7* (1941): 47–48.

37. Palmer, C. E. and Edwards, P. Q.: The Histoplasmin Skin Test. In *Histoplasmosis* (Sweaney, H. C., Ed.). Springfield, Charles C Thomas, Publisher, 1960.

38. Menges, R. W.: The Histoplasmin Skin Test in Animals. J. Amer. Vet. Med. Ass., *119* (1951): 69–71.

39. Saslaw, S., Maurice, G. E., and Cole, C. R.: Experimental Histoplasmosis in Large Animals. J. Lab. Clin. Med., *46* (1955): Abs. 96, P. 948.

40. Robinson, V. and McVickar, D. L.: Pathology of Spontaneous Canine Histoplasmosis. A Study of Twenty-one Cases. Amer. J. Vet. Res., *13* (1952): 214–219.

41. Smith, H. A. and Jones, T. C.: *Veterinary Pathology.* 3rd edition, Philadelphia, Lea & Febiger, 1966.

42. Straub, M. and Schwarz, J.: General Pathology of Human and Canine Histoplasmosis. Amer. Rev. Resp. Dis., *82* (1960): 528–541.

43. Pine, L.: Morphological and Physiological Characteristics of Histoplasma Capsulatum. In *Histoplasmosis* (Sweaney, H. C., Ed.). Springfield, Charles C Thomas, Publisher, 1960.

44. Procknow, J. J.: The Pathogenesis of Histoplasmosis in Animals. In *Histoplasmosis* (Sweaney, H. C., Ed.). Springfield, Charles C Thomas, Publisher, 1960.

45. Pine, L., Boone, C. J. and McLaughlin, D.: Antigenic Properties of the Cell Wall and Other Fractions of the Yeast Form of *Histoplasma capsulatum.* J. Bact., *91* (1966): 2158–2168.

46. Meleney H. E.: Toxoplasmosis Mistaken for Histoplasmosis Amer. J. Trop Med., *25* (1945): 163.

47. Vanbreuseghem, R.: *Histoplasma duboisii* and African Histoplasmosis. Mycologia, *45* (1953): 803–816.

48. Wilson, J. W. and Plunkett, O. A.: *The Fungous Diseases of Man.* Berkeley, University of California Press, 1965.

49. Zeidberg, L. D., Ajello, L., Dillon, A., and Runyon, L. C.: The Isolation of Histoplasma Capsulatum from Soil. Amer. J. Public Health, *42* (1952): 930–935.

50. Klite, P. D. and Diercks, F. H.: Histoplasma Capsulatum in Fecal Contents and Organs of Bats in the Canal Zone. Amer. J. Trop. Med., *14* (1965): 433–439.

51. Tosh, F. E., Balhuizen, J., Yates, J. L., and Brasher, C. A.: Primary Cutaneous Histoplasmosis. Arch. Intern. Med., *114* (1964): 118–119.

52. Ajello, L., Hosty, T. S., and Palmer, J.: Bat Histoplasmosis in Alabama. Amer. J. Trop. Med., *16* (1967) 329–331.

CHAPTER 9 | Blastomycosis

Blastomycosis, caused by the dimorphic fungus *Blastomyces dermatitidis*, is a granulomatous and suppurative disease of various animals and man. It originates from a primary pulmonary focus and may disseminate to the body organs or skin. Dogs are the most susceptible of the lower animals.

HISTORY, GEOGRAPHIC DISTRIBUTION AND PREVALENCE

Gilchrist,[1] in 1894, first described and reported blastomycosis in a human patient, and the infection is sometimes called Gilchrist's disease. In 1898, Gilchrist and Stokes[2] reported another case and named the causative fungus *Blastomyces dermatitidis*. Infections in man have also been called "the Chicago disease," because many of the early cases were discovered in that general vicinity.

The name North American blastomycosis became popular for the disease in both animals and man due to the early belief that infections were confined to North America. Recent information, however, indicates a much wider geographic distribution and renders that name invalid. Confusion has resulted also from the use of the name "European blastomycosis" for infections caused by *Cryptococcus neoformans*. Both the known geographic limits and the nomenclature of many mycotic diseases have undergone many changes, as the knowledge of medical mycology has progressed. It has been recommended that the name "blastomycosis," although not botanically correct, be reserved for the disease caused by the fungus *Blastomyces dermatitidis*.

If infections caused by the *Candida* species, *Cryptococcus neoformans* and *Paracoccidioides brasiliensis* were consistently referred to as candidiasis, cryptococcosis and paracoccidioidomycosis, respectively, there would be no confusing ambiguities and cause for misunderstanding. In the past, and even today, the term blastomycosis has been used in reference to any infection caused by a yeast. For the sake of clarity the imprecise use of the name blastomycosis should be abandoned.[3]

During the half century following the original discovery, blastomycosis in man was usually described as occurring in two main forms, cutaneous and systemic. The cutaneous form of the disease was generally believed to result from primary infection of the skin. The more modern concept is that, in almost all cases, the lungs are the primary focus of infection. Basing their conclusions on the tissues involved, most authorities now classify the disease in man as primary pulmonary, systemic or chronic cutaneous.[4,5] The two latter forms occur following hematogenous dissemination from the primary site.

The first reference to blastomycosis in dogs is credited to Meyer, in Philadelphia in 1912. However, only the title of his paper was published.[6] Herzog, in collaboration with MacLane,[7] described the histopathologic changes in the lungs of a canine case in Chicago in 1916. Martin and Smith[8] recorded a case of pulmonary canine blastomycosis in North Carolina in 1936 and were the first to prove the diagnosis by culture of the causative fungus.

Foshay and Madden[9] first described generalized blastomycosis in a dog in Ohio in 1942. The disease was rapidly fulminating with death occurring in a matter of weeks after the owner observed "bumps on the skin." The authors stated that abscesses were evident in the skin and subcutaneous tissues over much of the body. At necropsy they observed abscesses in the lungs, liver and spleen with pneumonic consolidation, splenomegaly and hepatomegaly. Small abscesses in the lymph nodes, kidneys and intestines, and pus in the aqueous humor of one of the eyes were also described.[9] This apparently is the first recorded instance of eye involvement in a dog infected by *Blastomyces dermatitidis*. The diagnosis was culturally confirmed. Another disseminated canine case, proved by culture, was disclosed in 1942 by Madsen from New York.[10]

Anthony[11] reported a case of pulmonary canine blastomycosis in 1945. His case, together with another (both in North Carolina), which was disseminated and rapidly fatal, was described by Seibold in 1946.[12] Cutaneous blastomycosis was reported in a dog in Iowa by Saunders in 1948.[13] He assumed that the infection disseminated after surgery on an affected ear. Oral, skin and subcutaneous lesions appeared soon after removal of the aural growth, and the subject died approximately three weeks following the surgery. Thoracic radiographs had not been made, nor was permission for a postmortem examination obtained. The author discussed the possi-

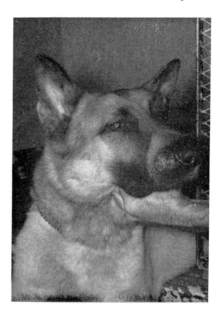

Fig. 9–1. Lesion on muzzle of four-year-old German shepherd with blastomycosis. Submandibular and cervical lymph nodes are markedly enlarged.

bility of a primary focus in the lungs. This now seems the more probable source of the infection.

Prior to 1950, only ten cases of canine blastomycosis had been described in the literature. However, several unreported cases had been discovered in the Chicago area, and these were included in a review by Ramsey and Carter[14] in which they described additional cases in Iowa. They summarized the salient clinical characteristics of 14 cases. All of the cases, with one exception on which a necropsy was not performed, had lung lesions.[13] Skin lesions were evident in four of the dogs, and bone or joint involvement was evident in three.

In the decade of the 1950s, it became evident that the prevalence of blastomycosis in dogs was greater than was indicated by the reports of the previous years. In 1954 Menges and co-workers, reporting seven cases in Kentucky, made the interesting observation that many of the affected dogs radiographically showed an enlargement at the base of the trachea.[15] At necropsy, the masses were found to be infected lymph nodes which had become greatly enlarged. Enlargement of the lymph nodes at the base of the trachea had been observed by Robinson and Schell[16] in a case they reported in 1951.

Newberne and associates[17] reported two cases from Alabama, and one each from Mississippi and Louisiana. One of their cases was diagnosed antemortem from biopsy of an affected lymph node. Another, discovered at necropsy, was thought to be a nonfatal pulmonary infection. The dog had been euthanized because of debility due to a fractured mandible and a malignancy.

By 1960, more than one hundred additional cases had been recorded. Menges[18] reviewed the clinical signs, tissues affected, and geographic distribution of many of these cases. He detailed the age distribution of 96 proven cases and discussed an epizootic that had occurred in Alabama. Menges and colleagues,[19] in 1965, reviewed the results of some previous studies and added their observations on 79 cases in Arkansas. They mapped a revised suspected endemic area for blastomycosis in North America, and showed the distribution of 263 canine cases.

The endemic area, based on present knowledge, includes the eastern half of the United States and the southern portion of Canada. Much of the area within the United States overlaps the endemic area for histoplasmosis. Texas has the dubious distinction of having endemic areas for blastomycosis, histoplasmosis and coccidioidomycosis. This presents difficult differential problems for veterinarians in that state. Recently three pets, each with a different systemic mycotic disease, were hospitalized simultaneously at the Texas A. & M. University clinic.

Several indisputable autochthonous cases of *Blastomyces dermatitidis* infection in man were reported from different areas in Africa in 1964. Prior reports of cases from Venezuela and Mexico were cited recently by Ajello who advanced the possibility of the occurrence of *B. dermatitidis* in Latin America.[3] It seems reasonable to expect reports of blastomycosis in animals in the future from these—and perhaps other—areas.

Skin testing and soil isolation studies have not been as productive in establishing endemic areas for blastomycosis as with some other fungus diseases. *Blastomyces dermatitidis* has only rarely been found in nature, and the skin test has not been adequately used or evaluated. When the natural habitat of the fungus is found in nature, there will, no doubt, be further changes in the concepts of its distribution.

Canine blastomycosis has been diagnosed most frequently in the Mississippi and

Ohio River valleys of the United States. With only one exception, all the states bordering those rivers have had reported cases. In certain areas of Kentucky and Arkansas, a comparatively high prevalence of cases was found as a result of intensive mycotic disease studies.[15,19]

Other than in the dog, blastomycosis of animals is indeed rare. One case of cutaneous infection has been reported in a horse,[20] and one systemic infection has been described in a captive sea lion.[21] Only six feline cases have been disclosed.[22,23,39]

CLINICAL SIGNS AND PATHOLOGY

Dogs with blastomycosis display a wide range of clinical signs related to the tissues or organs affected. The disease in dogs, in common with other mycotic diseases, is similar to infections in man. There are, however, some notable variations. Ocular lesions in man are apparently quite rare. They are only casually mentioned in recent medical mycology texts.[4,5] Eye lesions, many of which progress to blindness, are evident in approximately 20 percent of canine cases. Greatly enlarged mediastinal and bronchial lymph nodes, which appear on radiographs as a dense mass at the bifurcation of the trachea, are quite common in dogs. Conant[24] mentions that enlargement of the mediastinal nodes in man is a striking feature only in rare instances. In man, destructive lesions of the ribs and vertebrae are frequent.[5] Bone lesions and lameness are observed in dogs less frequently than are ocular lesions. The majority of canine cases occur in young dogs; in contrast, most human cases occur between the ages of 25 to 69 years.[18] Human males are afflicted much more frequently than females, the ratio is as high as fifteen to one in some studies. The incidence in dogs is more nearly equal between the sexes.

The most striking difference in the disease of man and dog is in those cases with skin lesions. Chronic localized cutaneous blastomycosis is the most common form observed in man. Seen first as a cutaneous lesion, it apparently remains limited to the skin throughout a chronic course extending over many years.[4] This form of the human disease, thought by most authorities to represent localization in the skin following dissemination from a primary pulmonary focus, is quite rare in dogs.

Dogs with cutaneous lesions are not destined to have a long, chronic illness. Skin and subcutaneous nodal lesions in dogs usually indicate dissemination to other parts of the body and, in many cases, represent an advanced stage of the disease. Writers almost invariably define blastomycosis as a chronic disease. This description does not seem as applicable to the disease in animals as in man.

There is reasonable doubt that a benign or inapparent form of blastomycosis occurs in animals. References to nonfatal and recovered cases can be found.[17,22,25,26] but they are indeed rare, as are reports of benign infections.[19,27] Admittedly, adequate surveys have not been made; but until wholly dependable diagnostic antigens are available, the occurrence of a mild respiratory form of blastomycosis (as has been well-established in coccidioidomycosis and histoplasmosis) will remain speculative.

Canine blastomycosis is characterized by pyrexia and debility, with cough, dyspnea and cutaneous lesions as the outstanding signs. The lungs, lymph nodes and skin are the tissues most frequently involved. Cutaneous ulcers, furuncles, and subcutaneous abscesses, without regional adenopathy, are common initial signs.[28] A history of cough and dyspnea, persistent or recurrent, followed by cutaneous lesions, should immediately alert the clinician to the possibility of blastomycosis.

Ocular lesions, many of which progress to blindness, are common. Eye disorders may be the initial signs observed.[29] Eye and nasal discharges, occurring concurrently, are frequent manifestations.

Swollen joints, testicles and lymph glands, though not consistent visible signs, are occasionally observed. The affected lymph nodes may be draining. Lameness and incoordination may be apparent. Dysphagia may occur due to compression of the esophagus, by enlarged lymph nodes, at its proximity to the bifurcation of the trachea.

The gross changes seen at necropsy may be limited to the lungs and adjacent lymph nodes. Depending upon the extent of the infection, the lungs may have few or many nodules of solidification, either circumscribed or diffuse. Robbins[30] has described lungs which contained thousands of nodules, 1 to 10 mm. in diameter, which were irregular, firm and greyish yellow. The nodules may appear caseated. However, upon incision, many of the cut surfaces will yield purulent exudate.

Enlargement of the bronchial and mediastinal lymph nodes is common in canine blastomycosis. Variations from slight enlargement to nodular masses of neoplastic appearance may be seen. The mass may compress the large bronchi and partially obliterate the lumen.[16]

In the more generalized form of the disease, lesions are frequently found in many body organs. Nodules may be seen in the liver, spleen and kidneys. Males may have visible lesions in the prostate or testicles. Ovarian lesions are less frequently observed, due, at least in part, to the common practice of oophorectomy. The intestine is usually spared.

Microscopically, the lesions of canine blastomycosis are characteristically granulomatous and suppurative. Typically, the proliferative lesions are composed of small granulomata with circumscribed accumulations of epithelioid type histiocytes arranged in circular fashion. Lymphocytes, either diffusely distributed or more commonly concentrated toward the periphery, are prominent. Lesser numbers of macrophages and occasional multinucleated cells of the foreign body type may be found. The fungus cells are found in the central necrotic areas and frequently within the cytoplasm of the giant cells also. Caseation necrosis may occur.

The suppurative lesions consist primarily of polymorphonuclear leucocytes and macrophages. Large numbers of organisms may be found concentrated in the abscesses or scattered throughout the surrounding tissue. Although some fibroblasts are recognizable, there is little tendency toward encapsulation of the lesions. Calcification is infrequent.[31] Combinations of both exudative and proliferative tissue reactions are found frequently.

Blastomyces dermatitidis appears in the lesions, free or in macrophages, as spherical or oval yeastlike cells which range from 5 to 20 μ in diameter. There is a characteristic sharply defined wall of sufficient thickness to give a "doubly contoured" appearance. If stained by hematoxylin and eosin, the protoplasm is usually very prominent, appears granular, and is generally pulled away from the cell wall, leaving a clear space. Several nuclei per cell may be demonstrated with special nuclear stains. Single budding cells are characteristic, with the daughter cell or bud attached by a broad base to the mother cell. However, multiple budding occurs occasionally. Stains for bound glycogen (PAS, Bauer, Gridley stains) will stain the outer wall of the organism selectively, differentiating it more clearly from the surrounding tissue. Some pathologists prefer sections stained with Gomori meth-

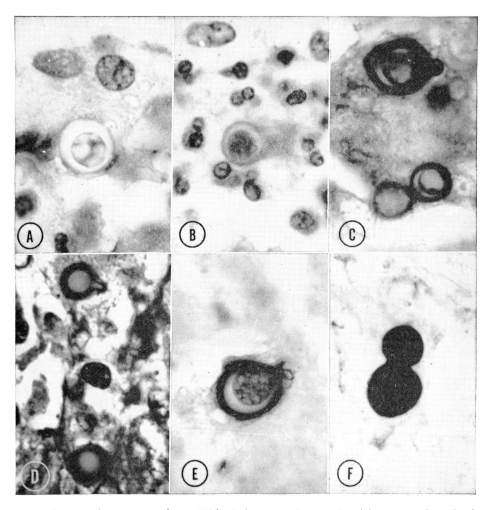

Fig. 9–2. *Blastomyces dermatitidis* in lung sections stained by several methods and photographed at × 1350. 663116. **A. H & E.** In the process of fixation the protoplasm has been pulled away from the lightly stained rigid cell wall, leaving an artificially produced clear space. The fungus cell is within a giant cell. (57–9202). **B.** Another field in slide described in **A.** The protoplasm is well-stained with hematoxylin and is multinucleate. Observe the large bud which is not in the same plane as the parent cell. (57–9199). **C. PAS.** The deep red of the stain appears black in the picture. One cell shows the beginning of a bud and the double cell is the final stage of budding. The fungus cells are within a giant cell. (57–9207). **D.** Another field from the section shown in **C.** Observe the wide opening between the parent cell and the bud in the fungus cell, upper field. The cell in the lower field demonstrates a slight protrusion of the wall where budding was about to take place. (57–9731). **E.** Gridley fungus stain of a budding cell. The purplish red wall appears black in the picture. The well-stained protoplasm has, as the result of fixation, pulled away from the wall leaving a well-defined clear space. (57–9205). **F.** Gomori methenamine-silver stain of a budding cell. The cell wall is so deeply silvered that no internal details are shown. (57–9734). (Emmons, Binford and Utz, Medical Mycology, courtesy of Lea & Febiger)

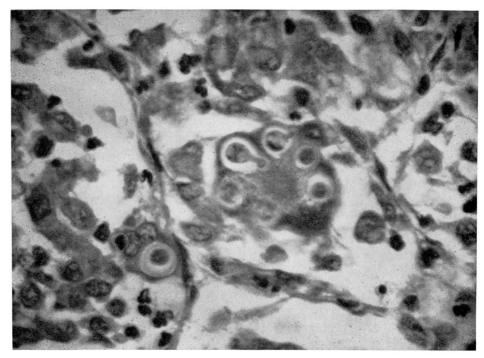

Fig. 9–3. *Blastomyces dermatitidis* in lung of dog. (Courtesy of Dr. C. H. Bridges)

enamine-silver in which the fungal cell walls are stained black and are easily distinguished.

Since there is some variation in the morphologic features of *Blastomyces dermatitidis*, the disease may be misdiagnosed on the basis of histopathologic studies alone. For example, the disease may be difficult to differentiate from histoplasmosis when small forms of *B. dermatitidis* are present, or when large forms of *Histoplasma capsulatum* or *H. duboisii* occur. If budding forms of *B. dermatitidis* are not seen, the cells may be mistaken for the immature sporangia of *C. immitis*. *Paracoccidioides brasiliensis* cells with only one bud may be mistaken for *B. dermatitidis* which furthermore may occasionally show multiple budding. Even *Cryptococcus neoformans*, in the absence of a capsule, may be mistaken for this organism.[32,33] Experienced pathologists usually can identify the organism with confidence; however, in view of the many similarities to other yeastlike organisms seen in tissue, unequivocal proof is by cultural confirmation.

Paracoccidioidomycosis, a disease similar in many respects to "North American blastomycosis," has been called "South American blastomycosis." The etiologic agent, however, is the dimorphic fungus *Paracoccidioides brasiliensis* and, therefore, the disease is more correctly called paracoccidioidomycosis. There are many similarities between *Paracoccidioides brasiliensis* and *Blastomyces dermatitidis*—both in culture and in the diseases they produce. The histopathologic reactions to both fungi are remarkably similar, both eliciting characteristic granulomatous reactions combined with suppurative inflammation. The tissue form of *P. brasiliensis* is a thick-walled yeastlike cell which produces single or multiple buds. In contrast to *B. dermatitidis*, the buds have a narrow point of attachment to the mother cell. If only one bud is produced, it may be difficult to differentiate *P. brasiliensis* from *B. dermatitidis* unless the manner of attachment is clearly seen. A search for the more characteristic multiple budding forms must be sought in most cases.

Paracoccidioidomycosis has been reported only in man, however, it seems reasonable to expect that it may eventually be found in animals also. The disease is geographically limited to Latin America with the majority of cases reported from Brazil. In a few instances, paracoccidioidomycosis ("South American blastomycosis") has been diagnosed in the United States. In all cases but one, however, the patients had visited or come from endemic areas of Latin America. The exception was a recent case in California. The subject had lived in California for 17 years and had visited Mexico—but not an area known to be endemic.[36] Several excellent references are available to the student with further interest in this disease.[4,5,33]

LABORATORY DIAGNOSIS

A laboratory diagnosis of blastomycosis can often be given provisional support from examination of clinical materials. In cutaneous infections, pus may be expressed from microabscesses in the periphery of skin lesions. The area should be thoroughly treated with iodine first and then alcohol. Pus scraped or withdrawn from subcutaneous abscesses often contains the fungus in great numbers.

In disseminated infections without skin lesions, pleural and peritoneal exudates should be requested. Spinal fluid and needle biopsy specimens from the liver may be rewarding. Urine may be useful, and if hematuria or pyuria are evident, genitourinary infection should be considered. In this case, prostatic secretions should be obtained from males.

It is often difficult to obtain satisfactory clinical specimens in primary pulmonary infections. In such cases, Tiegland culture tubes may be useful for obtaining tracheal exudates for examination and culture.

Direct Microscopic Examination

Body fluids and pus should be freshly obtained and examined unstained with subdued light in order to observe clearly the characteristic fungal cells. Pus may require dilution with water or hydroxide solution if it is dense or mucinous. (Staining is usually not desirable, since stained fungal cells are difficult to differentiate from lymphocytes.) *Blastomyces dermatitidis* occurs as thick-walled, round or oval cells 8 to 15 μ in diameter. Occasionally the cells may be as small as 5 μ, rarely as large as 30 μ in diameter. Cells with attached buds should be sought. A young bud has a wall much thinner than that of the parent, but the point of attachment may be as wide as the bud. The typical thick wall develops as the bud matures and the wide attachment persists.

If characteristic budding cells are not found, a saline moistened specimen may be ringed with petrolatum and topped with a cover slip. Incubate at room temperature. Within a few hours the cells may produce single germ tubes. In contrast, *Coccidioides immitis*, when similarly treated, produces several germ tubes from each spherule.

Culture

Clinical materials should be inoculated onto media containing cycloheximide and chloramphenicol. These antibiotics suppress most fungal and bacterial contaminants, but allow most pathogenic fungi to grow at room temperature. Because some of the pathogenic fungi are nutritionally fastidious, enriched media such as brain heart infusion agar or blood agar should be used in parallel with Sabouraud's agar containing these antibiotics. Growth is slow when isolating the organisms from clinical material, and visible growth may not appear for 10 to 14 days. If mycelial growth—morphologically suggestive of *B. dermatitidis*—appears, confirm by transferring to large screw-cap tubes of brain heart infusion agar or blood agar (without antibiotics) for 37° C. incubation to obtain the yeast form.

Room temperature cultures may first appear moist and glabrous or membranous, however, a fluffy or downy aerial mycelium soon develops which is initially white, but it often becomes cream-colored to light brown. Microscopic examination reveals the hyphae to be regularly septate. Characteristic smooth-walled conidia are borne along the sides of the hyphae and on the tips of short lateral branches (conidiophores). They are three to five μ in diameter and are round, oval or pyriform. They are thin-walled at first and the contents appear homogenous. Later they enlarge, the wall thickens and the contents appear granular.

The parasitic (yeastlike or tissue) form of *Blastomyces dermatitidis* can be maintained in vitro by incubation at 37° C. The tissue form will grow on simple media, but better growth results if it is grown on BHI agar or a blood agar medium. Media containing cycloheximide or chloramphenicol should not be used when incubating

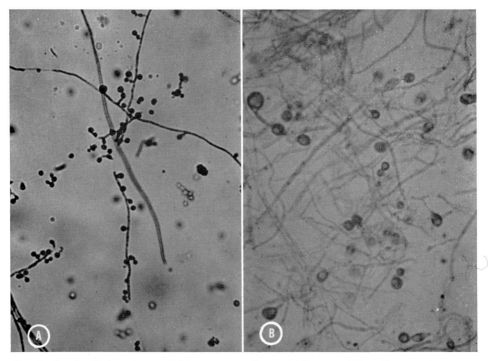

Fig. 9–4. **A.** Slide culture of *Blastomyces dermatitidis.* ✕ 400. Cotton Blue stain.
B. Slide mount of *B. dermatitidis* in Cotton Blue stain.

at 37° C. These antibiotics, at this temperature, suppress the growth of the tissue forms of the systemic fungi. *B. dermatitidis* grows slowly, producing cream-colored to tan, waxlike colonies in 10 to 14 days. The surface often becomes wrinkled with age. All culture tubes, incubated at 25° or 37° C., should be held for 30 days before they are discarded as negative.

Microscopically, the cells are identical to those found in tissue. However, a greater tendency toward multiple budding occurs in vitro than in vivo. The most distinguishing feature is the wide point of attachment between the daughter and parent cell. The wide attachment is apparent with young buds; this characteristic is retained by older buds in which the attachment may have a diameter of four to five μ.

Conversion of the yeastlike form of the fungus to the mycelial form can be readily accomplished by incubating the subculture at room temperature. The reciprocal conversion results from transfers of mycelium to fresh media and incubation at 37° C. The addition of sterile serum or broth to the surface of agar slants in screw-cap tubes will prevent excessive drying. Saline suspensions of mycelium can be injected intraperitoneally into mice for conversion to the tissue form.

There are a number of saprophytic fungi which resemble the mycelial form of *B. dermatitidis*. It is therefore essential to cultivate the fungus in its converted yeastlike "tissue form" to confirm its identification.

Pathogenicity Tests

Intraperitoneal injection of one ml. of a heavy saline suspension of either mycelial or yeast form cells will usually produce a demonstrable infection in mice. More extensive infections result from the addition of five-percent gastric mucin to the inoculum.[34] Clinical materials should be treated with antibacterial antibiotics prior to inoculation to prevent bacteria from killing the experimental animal. If the experimental mice survive, they should be sacrificed after three weeks.

Gross lesions are usually confined to the peritoneal cavity. Caseous material, pus or nodules may be found on the abdominal viscera. Nodules may be present in the lungs in extensive infections. Microscopic examination of fresh preparations shows the characteristic thick-walled, single-budded forms of *Blastomyces dermatitidis*.

Experimental infections have been produced in guinea pigs, monkeys, dogs, a sheep and a horse.[16] The disease syndrome which resulted depended upon the route of inoculation. Subcutaneous inoculations of a pure culture produced localized lesions in the horse, and intravenous injections resulted in a systemic infection in the dog. Subcutaneous injections of mycelia into monkeys resulted only in chronic granulomatous skin lesions. When several dogs were given injections similar to those received by the monkeys, they developed granulomatous skin lesions only which healed spontaneously in from four to eight weeks.

Immunology

As was previously stated, the clinical syndrome of blastomycosis in dogs differs in many respects from the disease in man. Generally speaking, the disease runs a much faster course in dogs, and it seems safe to hypothesize that they lack the ability to develop immunologic barriers to infection with *Blastomyces dermatitidis*. Adequate proof for the existence of a benign form of the disease in dogs is

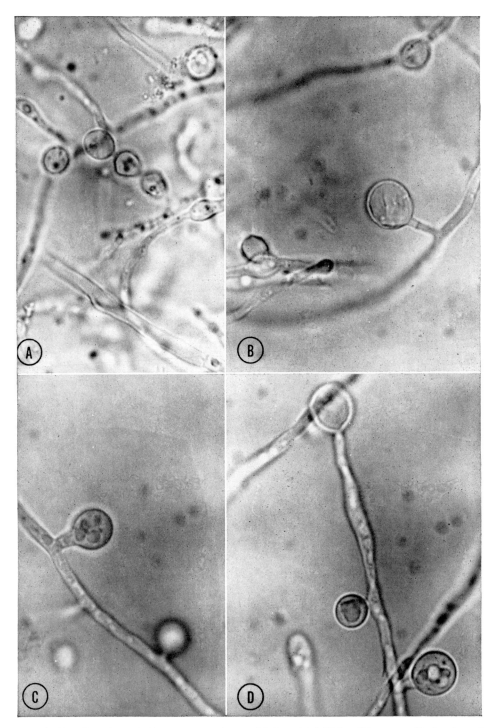

Fig. 9–5. Conidia of *Blastomyces dermatitidis*. × 1575. (Emmons, Binford and
Utz, Medical Mycology, courtesy of Lea & Febiger)

lacking, and this gives support to this hypothesis. Only very rarely do dogs develop the chronic cutaneous form of blastomycosis which is the most common form in man. The cellular reaction engendered in the skin of man by *B. dermatitidis* is tremendous; a dense infiltrate consisting of thousands of lymphocytes and plasma cells for every fungus cell is contained beneath an epidermis so strongly stimulated that it closely resembles a carcinoma (pseudoepitheliomatous hyperplasia). This phenomenon certainly suggests a high degree of resistance and indicates that the skin also participates in the immunologic reaction.[4]

The foregoing points have been stressed because they may, in part, explain the difficulty in obtaining and interpreting wholly satisfactory skin and serologic tests. Blastomycin is a sterile filtrate from cultures of the mycelial form of *Blastomyces dermatitidis* grown on liquid synthetic medium and is used to determine "skin-test sensitivity." Various blastomycins, made from several strains of the fungus, have been used in skin-test surveys for the disease in dogs.[19] The antigens were used in different dilutions for evaluation. Results of the limited experiments indicate that blastomycin is less specific than histoplasmin and coccidioidin and is therefore less useful as a diagnostic aid.

Blastomycin* is now commercially available as a standardized product for use in man. The manufacturer recommends that for use in dogs it be concentrated to 10 times the strength used in man. The antigen is injected and the test interpreted as was described for histoplasmin in Chapter 8 on histoplasmosis. The limitations described for the histoplasmin skin test are also applicable to the use of blastomycin. Cross-reactivity problems can be alleviated partially by testing with both antigens. The specific reaction should be stronger than the nonspecific one.

Of the serologic tests, the complement fixation (CF) test has been shown to be of most value. The test in its present form, however, is less useful in diagnosis than the CF tests for coccidioidomycosis or histoplasmosis.[33] Serums positive to other mycotic diseases will cross-react, but the major cross-reaction occurs between histoplasmosis and blastomycosis. Simultaneous tests with the different antigens should be run for both diseases. The homologous serum should have a higher titer. Unfortunately, this is not always the result. Dogs with proven blastomycosis have, in some cases, been shown to have higher titers for histoplasmosis.[19]

The difficulty in interpreting serologic test results was explained partially in a study by Kaufman and Kaplan.[35] They demonstrated five antigenic fractions which were either independent or were common fractions between the yeast and mycelial forms of both *Blastomyces dermatitidis* and *Histoplasma capsulatum*. The yeast forms of these two fungi have three common antigenic components. Each contains a specific antigen which can be separated by adsorption techniques. However, multiple adsorptions tend to make experimental antiglobulins anticomplementary, thus limiting its use. Similarly, the Ouchterlony agar-gel procedure has its own limitations in the analysis of adsorbed fungal antiglobulins. The report of Kaufman and Kaplan poses an interesting question. Does the cross-reactivity of *B. dermatitidis* and *H. capsulatum* indicate cross-protection?

The problems with the various immunologic tests make it quite apparent that they should not be used solely for diagnosis. They are useful aids if correlated with clinical, laboratory and radiologic findings.

* Parke, Davis & Company, Detroit, Michigan.

DIFFERENTIAL DIAGNOSIS

Canine blastomycosis may simulate respiratory diseases of bacterial and viral etiology. Cases with cerebral and meningeal involvement must be distinguished from distemper. Those with respiratory signs and ocular lesions may resemble infectious canine hepatitis. Nocardiosis, and other pulmonary and systemic mycotic infections, should be considered. Diarrhea is rarely a part of the clinical syndrome in canine blastomycosis. This feature is an aid in differentiating blastomycosis from histoplasmosis and coccidioidomycosis.

Those cases with cutaneous involvement may simulate a number of pustular, suppurative and granulomatous dermatoses, including those with allergic manifestations. Secondary bacterial invasion is common, and a patient search may be required to find the fungus in clinical material.

Radiographic examinations may be a valuable diagnostic and differential aid. A dense mass at the bifurcation of the trachea, either with or without local or diffuse pulmonary consolidation, is often present. This finding, together with a history of a chronic cough and the presence of ocular or cutaneous lesions, is highly suggestive of blastomycosis.

EPIDEMIOLOGY

The saprophytic existence of *Blastomyces dermatitidis* in soil was long suspected before it was finally proved[37] and confirmed.[38] Soil samples were treated with antibacterial antibiotics and were then injected intravenously into white Swiss mice via the tail vein. Indirect isolations were thus made from soil obtained from the earth floor of a tobacco stripping shed in Kentucky, and from soil associated with various animal habitats in Georgia. The tobacco stripping shed had previously housed a dog with blastomycosis. The animal habitats in Georgia included three chicken houses, a rabbit pen, a cattle loading ramp and a mule stall. This suggests that *B. dermatitidis* has a general association with animal habitats in contrast to the more specific ecologic relationship between *Histoplasma capsulatum* and the excreta of avian and chiropteran species.

Isolations cannot be made repeatedly from formerly "positive" soils, and the factors and conditions which allow *Blastomyces dermatitidis* to flourish in soil are still unknown. The fungus cannot be maintained for long periods in natural soils inoculated in the laboratory and held at room temperature. Ajello has studied the mycolytic activity of bacteria and actinomycetes on fungi in soil under natural conditions and in vitro. In his application of the biologic activity to the presence of *B. dermatitidis* in soil he stated, "All available clinical and epidemiological evidence strongly suggests that somewhere in nature an ecological niche exists that favors *B. dermatitidis*. We can be certain that through diligent field and laboratory work its natural habitat will eventually be discovered."[3]

It is generally accepted that man and animals become infected with *Blastomyces dermatitidis* (as with *Histoplasma capsulatum*) by inhalation of conidia from colonies of the mold growing as saprophytes in the soil or a similar substrate. A high percentage of all cases, in both animals and man, have evidence of pulmonary involvement.

Blastomycosis is not transmitted from individual to individual or from animals to man, but each individual or animal apparently acquires his infection independently and directly from nature.

TREATMENT

See Chapter 7, treatment of systemic mycoses, pp. 102–103.

REFERENCES

1. Gilchrist, T. C.: Protozoan Dermatitis. J. Cutan. Genito. Urin. Dis., *12* (1894): 496.
2. Gilchrist, T. C. and Stokes, W. R.: A Case of Pseudolupus Vulgaris Caused by Blastomyces. J. Exp. Med., *3* (1898): 53–78.
3. Ajello, L.: Comparative Ecology of Respiratory Mycotic Disease Agents. Bact. Rev., *31* (1967): 6–24.
4. Wilson, J. W. and Plunkett, O. A.: *The Fungous Diseases of Man.* Berkeley, University of California Press, 1965.
5. Emmons, C. W., Binford, C. H., and Utz, J. P.: *Medical Mycology.* 2nd edition, Philadelphia, Lea & Febiger, 1970.
6. Meyer, K. R.: Blastomycosis in Dogs. Proc. Path. Soc. Philadelphia, *15* (1912): 10.
7. Herzog, M. and MacLane, C. C.: Cases of Generalized Fatal Blastomycosis, Including One in a Dog. J. Infect. Dis., *19* (1916): 194–200.
8. Martin, D. S. and Smith, D. T.: The Laboratory Diagnosis of Blastomycosis. J. Lab. Clin. Med., *21* (1936): 1289–1296.
9. Foshay, L. and Madden, A. G.: The Dog as a Natural Host for *Blastomyces dermatitidis.* Amer. J. Trop. Med., *22* (1942): 565–569.
10. Madsen, D. E.: Some Studies of Three Pathogenic Fungi Isolated from Animals. Cornell Vet., *32* (1942): 383–389.
11. Anthony, C. H.: Canine Blastomycosis. Jen-Sal J., *28* (Nov.-Dec., 1945): 22.
12. Seibold, H. R.: Systemic Blastomycosis in Dogs. No. Amer. Vet., *27* (1946): 162–168.
13. Saunders, L. Z.: Cutaneous Blastomycosis in the Dog. No. Amer. Vet., *29* (1948): 650–652.
14. Ramsey, F. K. and Carter, G. R.: Canine Blastomycosis in the United States. J. Amer. Vet. Med. Ass., *120* (1952): 93–98.
15. Menges, R. W., McClellan, J. T., and Ausherman, R. J.: Canine Histoplasmosis and Blastomycosis in Lexington, Kentucky. J. Amer. Vet. Med. Ass., *124* (1954): 202–207.
16. Robinson, V. B. and Schell, F. G.: Blastomycosis in a Dog. A Case Report. No. Amer. Vet., *32* (1951): 555–558.
17. Newberne, J. W., Neal, J. E., and Heath, M. K.: Some Clinical and Microbiological Observations on Four Cases of Canine Blastomycosis. J. Amer. Vet. Med. Ass., *127* (1955): 220–223.
18. Menges, R. W.: Blastomycosis in Animals. Vet. Med., *55* (1960): 45–54.
19. Menges, R. W., Furcolow, M. L., Selby, L. A., Ellis, H. R., and Haberman, R. T.: Clinical and Epidemiologic Studies on Seventy-Nine Canine Blastomycosis Cases in Arkansas. Amer. J. Epidemiology, *81* (1965): 164–179.
20. Benbrook, E. A., Bryant, J. B. and Saunders, L. Z.: A Case of Blastomycosis in the Horse, J. Amer. Vet. Med. Ass., *112* (1948): 475–478.
21. Williamson, W. M., Lombard, L. S., and Getty, R. E.: North American Blastomycosis in a Northern Sea Lion. J. Amer. Vet. Med. Ass., *135* (1959): 513–515.
22. Easton, K. L.: Cutaneous North American Blastomycosis in a Siamese Cat. Canad. Vet. J., *2* (1961): 350–351.
23. Sheldon, W. G.: Pulmonary Blastomycosis in a Cat. Lab. Anim. Care, *16* (1966): 280–285.
24. Conant, N. F., Smith, D. T., Baker, R. D., Callaway, J. L., and Martin, D. S.: *Manual of Clinical Mycology.* 2nd edition, Philadelphia, W. B. Saunders Company, 1954.
25. Ausherman, R. J., Sutton, H. H., and Oakes, J. T.: Clinical Signs of Blastomycosis in Dogs. J. Amer. Vet. Med. Ass., *130* (1957): 541–542.
26. Selby, L. A., Haberman, R. T., Breshears, D. E., and Ellis, H. R.: Clinical Observations on Canine Blastomycosis. Vet. Med., *59* (1964): 1221–1228.
27. Selby, L. A., Menges, R. W., and Haberman, R. T.: Survey for Blastomycosis and Histoplasmosis Among Stray Dogs in Arkansas. Amer. J. Vet. Res., *28* (1967): 345–349.
28. Schwartzman, R. M., Fusaro, R. M., and Orkin, M.: Transmission of North American Blastomycosis. JAMA, *171* (1959): 2185–2189.

29. Wolf, G. F., Schwartzman, R. M., and Sautter, J. H.: Blastomycosis in a Dog. Vet. Med., *53* (1958): 595–600.
30. Robbins, E. S.: North American Blastomycosis in the Dog. J. Amer. Vet. Med. Ass., *125* (1954): 391–398.
31. Smith, H. A., Jones, T. C., and Hunt, R. D.: *Veterinary Pathology.* 4th edition, Philadelphia, Lea & Febiger, 1972.
32. Pappagianis, D.: Epidemiological Aspects of Respiratory Mycotic Infections. Bact. Rev., *31* (1967): 25–34.
33. Ajello, L., Georg, L. K., Kaplan, W., and Kaufman, L.: *Laboratory Manual for Medical Mycology.* Washington, U. S. Govt. Printing Office, 1963.
34. Strauss, R. and Kligman, A. M.: The Use of Gastric Mucin to Lower Resistance of Laboratory Animals to Systemic Fungus Infections. J. Infect. Dis., *88* (1951): 151–155.
35. Kaufman, L. and Kaplan, W.: Serologic Characterization of Pathogenic Fungi by Means of Fluorescent Antibodies. I. Antigenic Relationships Between Yeast and Mycelial Forms of *Histoplasma capsulatum* and *Blastomyces dermatitidis.* J. Bact., *85* (1963): 986–991.
36. Artiga, C. A.: A Case of South American Blastomycosis in California. Amer. J. Trop. Med., *17* (1968): 576–578.
37. Denton, J. F., McDonough, E. S., Ajello, L., and Ausherman, R. J.: Isolation of *Blastomyces dermatitidis* from Soil. Science, *133* (1961): 1126–1127.
38. Denton, J. F. and DiSalvo, A. F.: Isolation of *Blastomyces dermatitidis* from Natural Sites at Augusta, Georgia. Amer. J. Trop. Med., *13* (1964): 716–722.
39. Jasmin, A. M., Carroll, J. M., Baucom, J. N., and Beusse, D. O.: Systemic Blastomycosis in Siamese Cats, V.M./S.A.C., *64* (1969): 33–37.

CHAPTER 10 | Cryptococcosis

Cryptococcosis, caused by the yeastlike fungus *Cryptococcus neoformans*, is a subacute or chronic disease of man and various species of lower animals. The disease in dogs and cats is characterized by pulmonary and central nervous system involvement and/or by localized lesions of the oral and nasal mucosa. The infection in cattle usually involves mammary tissue and adjacent lymph nodes; horses manifest nasal discharges and respiratory distress associated with nasal granulomata.

HISTORY, GEOGRAPHIC DISTRIBUTION AND PREVALENCE

Although there are questionable prior reports,[1] most authorities credit the discovery and report of the first human case of cryptococcosis to Busse[2] and Buschke.[3] Independently in 1894–95, they reported the recovery of a yeastlike fungus from a case with skin and bone lesions. Busse referred to the disease as saccharomycosis hominis.

Sanfelice,[4] in 1894, isolated the same yeast from peach juice. He named the organism *Saccharomyces neoformans*, thus establishing priority to the species name *neoformans*. In 1895, he again isolated this yeastlike fungus from the lymph node of an ox (cited by Barron).[5] This apparently represents the first record of an infection in an animal. Vuillemin,[6] in 1901, found cryptococci in a pulmonary lesion in a pig. He recognized that the lack of ascospore formation differentiated the organism from the true yeasts, and he transferred it to the genus *Cryptococcus*. Klein,[7] also in 1901, described a pathogenic yeast he recovered from milk which subsequently was reported to be identical with strains of *C. neoformans* of human and plant origin.[8] Frothingham,[9] in 1902, described cryptococcosis in a horse. A myxomatous mass was found in the lung following a persistent nasal discharge of a year's duration.

Cryptococcus neoformans was found in several human cases in the early 1900s. In 1905, von Hansemann first observed the organism in association with meningitis. That now familiar clinical form of the human disease where central nervous system involvement is characteristic was first recognized in a living patient and reported by Verse in 1914.[10] The following year Stoddard and Cutler[11] reported additional cases and described the clinical and pathologic differences between cryptococcosis,

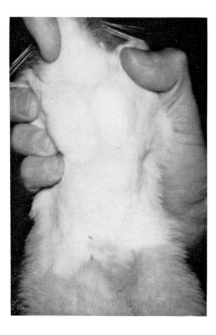

Fig. 10–1. Enlarged submandibular lymph
nodes in cat with cryptococcosis.

North American blastomycosis and other fungus infections. They named the
causative organism *Torula histolytica* because of an assumed "histolytic" action of
the organism in forming cysts in tissue. It is unfortunate that the name received so
much support. It lacks priority and is not supported by any taxonomic rule, and the
concept of histolytic activity on the part of this fungus is erroneous.[12]

Benham,[13] in 1935, after studying 22 strains of pathogenic cryptococci, cleared up
some of the confusion resulting from the use of the names blastomycosis and
European blastomycosis for the disease caused by the Busse-Buschke organism.
She evaluated its pathogenicity and suggested retaining the name *Cryptococcus
hominis* (originally proposed by Vuillemin) for the fungus. The consensus among
medical mycologists at present is that the most valid name, on the basis of usage
and priority, is *Cryptococcus neoformans*, with *Cryptococcus hominis* and *Torula
histolytica* falling into synonymy.[14]

Animal cases of cryptococcosis were reported only sporadically prior to 1950. A
mounting interest in animal mycoses developed at about that time, and reports
appeared with increasing frequency. Holzworth[15] first reported cryptococcosis in a
cat in 1952. The subject was a mature male which, at necropsy, was found to have
a generalized infection. In 1953, Holzworth and Coffin[16] reported a second feline
case in a mature spayed female with less extensive lesions. Both cats had histories
of chronic respiratory disorders of some duration. Okoshi and Hasegawa[28] recently
reported a generalized infection in a cat in Japan and included a world literature
review of feline cryptococcosis.

In 1953, Seibold and associates[17] first described cryptococcosis in a dog. Gross
postmortem changes were confined to the upper respiratory region. No gross
lesions were observed in the brain, but because the clinical signs were suggestive of
meningitis or encephalitis, the brain had been removed for histopathologic examination. Budding cells characteristic of *Cryptococcus neoformans* were found
within cystic cavities of the pia-arachnoid. The authors discussed the possibility of

the fungus having gained entrance to the brain by extension from the upper respiratory tract and middle ear. This point is noted here because complete agreement has not been reached by authors with regard to the primary infective focus and mode of dissemination of *C. neoformans*. Proponents of the theory that brain invasion can occur by direct extension of the infection from the nasopharynx can cite numerous cases in which lesions were found only in those sites. Wagner and co-workers[29] recently reviewed the literature on canine cryptococcosis and reported a case with meningoencephalitis in which *C. neoformans* gained entry into the CNS by extension of otitis externa. Some workers appear willing to concede that this type of brain invasion is possible; however, most believe that the usual primary focus is the lungs.

Wilson and Plunkett,[18] in their discussion of cryptococcosis in man, state their opinion as follows:

> Cryptococcosis is nearly always acquired by the inhalation of spores [cells] of the fungus along with terrestrial dust. Direct inoculation through the skin has been accepted as the portal of entry by some authors when reporting cases, but features that make this conclusion doubtful have usually been cited. Apparently the portal has sometimes been the oropharynx or the gastrointestinal tract.

Maddy summarized the opinions of several authorities when he stated that probably most cases result from inhalation of the fungus, which incites a pulmonary lesion that usually heals. It is likely that this is the end of most infections. However, spread to the central nervous system sometimes occurs with disastrous results. Many studies have concentrated on disseminated disease, thereby giving disproportionate emphasis on this phase of the disease.[19]

Cryptococcus neoformans is capable of primary invasion of the bovine mammary gland with subsequent severe mastitis and serious economic loss. Pounden and colleagues[20] reported the clinical aspects of an outbreak in which 106 cows were affected in a 235-cow herd in 1952. The pathologic aspects of the infections were reported by Innes and partners.[21] Emmons,[22] in another report, described the identifying features and characteristics of the organism. In 1953, Simon and fellow workers[23] reported another outbreak of bovine mastitis caused by *C. neoformans*. The initial source of the infection was not determined. Its spread was attributed to a herdsman's use of an antibiotic diluent which was contaminated with the fungus. (Since *C. neoformans* is not inhibited by antibacterial antibiotics, it can multiply readily in such media.) The authors stated that the organism was killed by standard milk pasteurization methods.

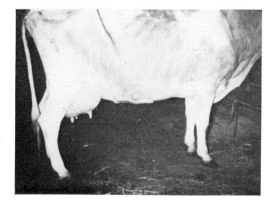

Fig. 10–2. Acute cryptococcal bovine mastitis. Cow became markedly dehydrated, and milk production ceased completely within 24 hours after onset of clinical signs.

Barron,[5] in 1953, reviewed the world literature on cryptococcosis of animals and noted, as in man, that central nervous system involvement is a common manifestation. Four of five cases in domestic cats, and all of five canine cases reviewed had central nervous system involvement. This observation was not applicable to the large domestic animals, for only one each of several bovine and equine cases were similarly involved. Pulmonary lesions and generalized infections were described both in conjunction with central nervous system involvement and independent of it. Barron's review, in addition to the animal species previously mentioned, included a case of cryptococcosis in the domestic pig, two in the cheetah, two in the Marmoset monkey and one in a small-toothed palm civet.

In the monograph of Littman and Zimmerman published in 1956,[14] the authors included an excellent chapter on cryptococcosis in animals. They cited the review of Barron and added other references to animal cases which included the monkey (sooty mangabey), fox, guinea pig and ferret.

Ajello,[24] in 1958, cited some early animal cases which were not included in the previously mentioned reviews. In a later publication, he added references to cases of cryptococcosis in a gazelle, goats, koalas, mink and a wallaby.[25]

Several interesting differences are apparent as regards *Cryptococcus neoformans* and its relationship to the dimorphic fungi that cause systemic diseases. *C. neoformans* exists in nature as a yeastlike fungus rather than in a mycelial form. Unlike the dimorphic pathogens, its saprophytic existence was discovered almost simultaneously with its capabilities as a virulent pathogen.

Clinically important infections are much more common in dogs with regard to diseases caused by the dimorphic fungus pathogens. Cryptococcosis, among the companion animal species, is at least equally important in cats. In total number of cases, bovine mammary infections outnumber the combined cases of all other lower animal species. Cryptococcosis in man is often associated with other diseases and has an association of statistical significance with lymphoblastomas, most often Hodgkin's disease and leukemia.[18] If a parallel condition is important in animal cases, it has not been discovered; however, a case of canine cryptococcosis with concomitant Hodgkin's disease was recently reported.[26]

Emmons and his co-authors[12] suggest the probability that cryptococcosis begins as a pulmonary disease with secondary hematogenous spread to skin, bones, abdominal viscera and especially to the central nervous system. Other authorities state that *Cryptococcus neoformans* has been cultured from the blood of infected persons, thus further indicating the possibility of hematogenous dissemination. In laboratory animals lymphatic spread has been observed also.[18]

Useful skin and serologic tests have not been available for prevalence surveys in animals or man, and absolute proof of a benign self-limited form of cryptococcosis must await the development of more specific antigens. It is certain that only a few of the total cases of cryptococcosis are now reported. Many animal cases are probably misdiagnosed—a very large number if a benign, self-limited form of the disease occurs. In any event, the disease is no doubt far more prevalent than is generally recognized.

CLINICAL SIGNS AND PATHOLOGY

There is a marked lack of consistency in the clinical signs exhibited by dogs and cats with cryptococcosis. Initially, infected individuals may show destructive granulomatous processes in the oral and pharyngeal mucosa. Similar lesions are sometimes seen involving nasal mucosa and turbinates, facial sinuses and adjacent osseous structures. Less commonly, lameness and, rarely, skin lesions are the first manifestation of *Cryptococcus neoformans* infection in the companion animal species. Eventually, most individuals will develop signs referable to central nervous system involvement. These may be somewhat vague (listlessness, pupil dilation, mild ataxia) or quite obvious as incoordination, circling and partial or complete blindness associated with locomotor disturbance. Some individuals show initial signs of CNS involvement; and although the primary infective focus was probably pulmonary, respiratory signs are usually not evident. Occasional cases of generalized infection occur in which the CNS is apparently spared. A marked or persistent pyrexia is not a feature of cryptococcosis.

The majority of cases of equine cryptococcosis have shown clinical signs of nasal "granulomas" only. Frothingham's case[9] was found, at necropsy, to have a myxomatous mass in the lung. Weidman[27] described a growth in the lip of a horse from which *Cryptococcus neoformans* was isolated. At necropsy, the animal was found to have had a generalized infection.

The clinical signs elicited by invasion of the bovine mammary gland by *Cryptococcus neoformans* are extremely variable. During an outbreak, the fungus has been isolated from samples when no visible changes were noted in either the gland or milk. The cases with visible signs vary from mild and transient swelling of one or more quarters of the udder to severe swelling and distention of the affected glands. The severe cases usually develop slowly. The glands are at first mildly affected, showing swelling and firmness in their dorsal parts. A slowly progressive involvement of the gland occurs during the next several days with eventual extreme swelling and firmness. The subcutaneous tissues of the udder and the area anteriorly adjacent usually become edematous. The severe clinical signs may persist for several weeks. On palpation, the supramammary lymph nodes frequently will be found to be enlarged.

Cows with mild infections often show no clinical signs of illness other than swelling of the affected glands. Those with severe infections apparently suffer considerable discomfort. They are reluctant to move and stand with the hindlegs abnormally spread. The body temperature is seldom elevated more than two degrees, and the characteristic clinical signs of severe bacterial mastitis (depression, anorexia, dehydration) are either absent or mild. Milk secretion gradually diminishes. In persistent cases, it ceases completely, even in apparently unaffected quarters.

Visible changes may not be apparent in the milk during the first days of the infection. Small white flakes may be noted first in the strip cup. In severe and persistent infections, watery serum containing flakes may characterize the secretion; more commonly the milk will appear grey-white, highly viscid and mucoid.

At necropsy, the gross lesions of cryptococcosis are not diagnostic. Lesions of the naso- or oropharynx may resemble a myxomatous neoplasm. In the lungs and abdominal viscera, the lesions usually appear as granulomatous nodules. In the former with progressive infection, the lesions may appear as miliary granulomas, small abscesses, or large solid or mucoid lesions of pneumonitis involving one or more lobes.

Macroscopic lesions of the central nervous system may be so minimal that the disease is not suspected as was noted in the original canine case reported by Seibold and associates.[17] The meningeal surface may appear edematous and feel slimy to the touch. In more obvious instances the meninges may be markedly reddened and thickened and obscure the underlying brain tissue.

The subarachnoid space may be distended with a greyish adherent exudate having a mucoid appearance which has been described as resembling tiny soap bubbles. When the exudate is present, the membranes are easily lifted off. In those cases in which the meningeal reaction is granulomatous, the membranes may adhere to the cortex. The surface of the cortex often has areas of fine dimpling, each dimple representing the site of a cystoid lesion containing the fungus cells.

Littman[14] has noted the similarity of the tissue reactions to *Cryptococcus neoformans* invasions in animals and man. Many writers have noted the relative paucity of both cellular and humoral reactions, especially in the nervous system. The description of Wilson and Plunkett is classic:

> Lesions of cryptococcosis are usually characterized by a startling mildness of the host's inflammatory response to the invading fungi; sometimes there is none at all, especially in brain involvement. In histopathologic study, this feature is revealed by an almost complete absence of cellular infiltrate in or around the masses of fungus cells, which accordingly appear almost as though in pure culture. A thin mantle of lymphocytes may be seen at the periphery. These masses constitute the so-called gelatinous tumors which, by their enlargement, exert enough pressure on the surrounding tissues simply to push them aside, a process earlier thought to be histolytic and thus responsible for an earlier name for the fungus (*Torula histolytica*). Large gelatinous cysts of this type, several centimeters in diameter, are frequently found in the lungs. In the central nervous system the subarachnoid space is often distended by similar gelatinous material resembling tiny soap bubbles, particularly over the base of the brain and in the region of the cerebellum, and cystic masses occur in the gray matter, sometimes near the surface, or deep in the region of the basal ganglia or the pons. The spinal meninges are often involved, but rarely the cord itself.[18]

In the brain and meninges, and occasionally in the lungs, the organisms grow and multiply rapidly, forming a cystic space occupied by the fungus cells the mucoid capsules of which account for the glistening appearance and slimy consistency encountered grossly. In such sites, the tissue reaction of the host is difficult to detect, although occasional macrophages with engulfed organisms may be found. In some sites, the organisms are less numerous and the tissue reaction much more profound. In lesions of this type, which may be adjacent to a cystic lesion, numerous endothelial cells with an admixture of lymphocytes are partially or completely surrounded by connective tissue. This granulomatous reaction is particularly prominent in some cases of cryptococcal mastitis but has been observed also in lesions of the brain, lung and other organs.[30]

Interestingly, in the outbreak of *Cryptococcus neoformans* mastitis described by Innes and associates,[21] the usual infection remained confined to the udder. In some cases the supramammary glands were infected. In a few cases, the external iliac or deep inguinal nodes were also affected. Only in one cow were cryptococcic lesions found in the lung, indicating the possibility of hematogenous dissemination. In no cases did infection of the nervous system occur.

Innes noted a considerable variation in the histologic picture of different affected quarters and, in some cases, in different parts of the same quarter. He related these

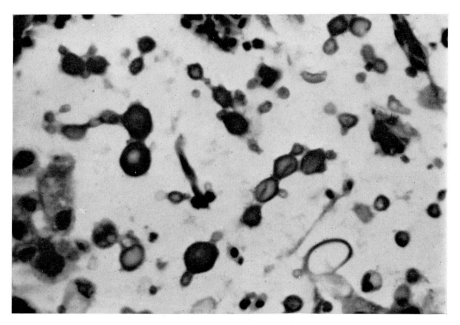

Fig. 10–3. *Cryptococcus neoformans* in lung of cat.

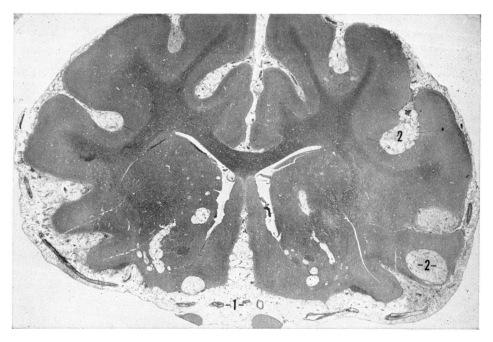

Fig. 10–4. Cryptococcosis brain of a cat. Large masses of organisms in leptomeninges (1) give them an edematous appearance and result in distention of depths of sulci (2). AFIP 523653. Contributor: Dr. John Mills. (Smith, Jones and Hunt, Veterinary Pathology, courtesy of Lea & Febiger)

differences to the severity and chronicity of the disease. In some areas the infection had resulted in the formation of large, irregular cysts containing little but the causative organism and presumably, in the fresh state, the mucoid secretion. In udders with lesions of a more chronic type, there was fibrous tissue proliferation in intra- and interlobular situations, and some foci contained epithelioid cells and thus were more granulomatous in nature.

Cryptococcus neoformans occurs in tissues as ovoid or spherical, thick-walled, yeastlike bodies which reproduce by the production of daughter cells (thin-walled at first) which are joined to the parent cell by a thin, narrow neck. A diligent search may be required to find typical budding cells because only a few will be cut by the microtome in the exact plane of mother and daughter cell attachment. The fungus cells vary greatly in size but are generally from five to ten μ in diameter, exclusive of their capsule. The gelatinous capsule may vary in thickness from one-half to five times the diameter of the cell. In hematoxylin and eosin stained sections, the cell wall and sometimes its contents are visible, but the capsule remains unstained giving the effect of a clear halo about the fungus cell. The capsule stains selectively (pink to red) with Mayer's mucicarmine stain. When stained by the periodic acid-schiff (PAS) method for glycogen, both the cell wall and capsule absorbs the rose to dark red stain.

So-called "germ-tubes" or elongated fingerlike projections which represent rudimentary pseudomycelium may be seen occasionally in tissues, but no true mycelium or any other fungal structures are developed by *Cryptococcus neoformans*. In localized infections, cryptococci may be small, thinly encapsulated and, when engulfed by giant cells and histiocytes, may resemble *Histoplasma capsulatum*. Mayer's mucicarmine stain readily differentiates the two organisms since *H. capsulatum* does not possess the pink-to-red staining mucinous capsular material of *C. neoformans*.[14]

LABORATORY DIAGNOSIS

The presence of nonpathogenic encapsulated cryptococci can be demonstrated in the air and upon the skin of animals, and the occurrence of these organisms as contaminants can confuse the identification of *Cryptococcus neoformans*. The fungus has been found in milk produced by apparently normal cows,[31] and it has been isolated from soil in many parts of the world.[25] The possibility of cryptococci as contaminants should be considered particularly when culturing nasal exudates from animals with myxomatous-like growths of the nasopharynx. The presence of *C. neoformans* does not necessarily constitute infection; and in most cases, in addition to culture, the organism should be demonstrated in tissues.

The combating of contaminants is a continuing problem in a diagnostic laboratory and is especially troublesome with many specimens from animals. Many isolations of *Cryptococcus neoformans* from man are obtained from sputum samples. This source of diagnostic material is not available to a veterinary mycology laboratory and, therefore, all other available specimens should be requested.

According to Littman,[14] the most important laboratory procedure in suspected cases of cryptococcal meningitis is examination of the spinal fluid. He further states that pathologic studies have revealed the frequency with which *Cryptococcus neoformans* may be found in the renal glomeruli and tubules, hepatic sinusoids, lymph nodes and bone marrow. He suggests that more frequent use of cultures of blood, urine and tissues, obtained by needle or surgical biopsy, would establish the

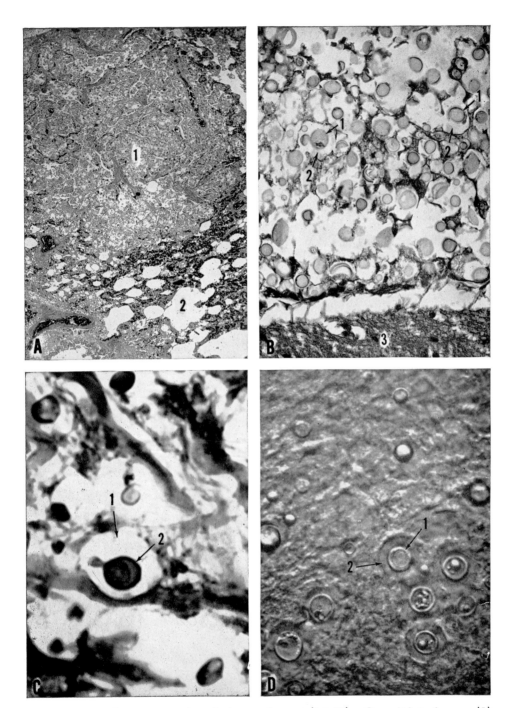

Fig. 10-5. Cryptococcosis. **A.** Lung of a cat (× 48). Consolidated area (1) filling and compressing alveoli (2). **B.** Organisms in pia mater of a cat (× 300). Note spherical organisms (1) surrounded by a wide, clear capsule (2). Cerebral cortex (3). AFIP 523563. Contributor: Dr. John Mills. **C.** Organisms in cat lung (× 1045), same case as **A.** Note wide unstained capsule (1) surrounding a budding organism (2). AFIP 324207. Contributor: Dr. Jean Holzworth. **D.** Unstained smear preparation viewed with phase contrast. Cell body (1) and capsule (2) (× 925). (Smith, Jones and Hunt, Veterinary Pathology, courtesy of Lea & Febiger)

diagnosis more often. As an example, he cited a case in which *C. neoformans* was recovered from the urine although repeated cultures of the blood and spinal fluid remained sterile.

Direct Microscopic Examination

Spinal fluid, milk, urine or other body fluids may be spread in a drop of India ink on a slide, covered with a cover slip, and examined under the microscope. If the specimen is too dense, the India ink may be diluted with a small drop of water. In the ink mounts, the mucinous capsule of cryptococci appears as a large transparent halo. With reduced light, the cell proper, with or without single buds, may be observed in the center of the capsule. Demonstration of encapsulated yeastlike cells in spinal fluid is prima facie evidence of cryptococcal meningitis, since no other encapsulated fungal species is capable of invading the nervous system of man or animals.[14]

If the initial search is unrewarding, the specimen may be centrifuged, and the concentrated sediment examined. Stained smears are of little value and may be misleading. The fungal cells shrink and become distorted in fixing, stain unevenly, and may be mistaken for blood cells or artifacts.

Culture

Cryptococcus neoformans differs culturally from the dimorphic systemic fungi in that it forms smooth, mucoid, yeastlike colonies when incubated at 20° C. and at 37° C. The fungus grows adequately on most ordinary laboratory media developing

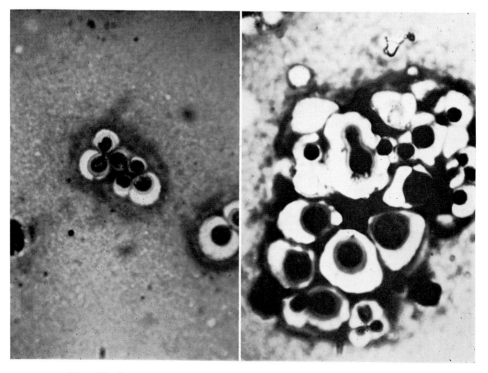

Fig. 10–6. *Cryptococcus neoformans* in mastitic bovine milk.

visible colonies within a few days. More abundant growth develops when a carbohydrate such as dextrose is incorporated in the medium. On Sabouraud dextrose agar (SDA) incubated at room temperature, soft and creamy, opaque, yeastlike colonies develop in three to five days. They appear smooth and glossy with a raised surface and smooth periphery. Microscopic examination at this stage of growth usually reveals that the capsules are not well-developed. After five to seven more days of incubation, the colonies become quite mucoid, develop an increased convexity, and are cream to tan in color. Characteristic budding cells with thick capsules may now be seen microscopically.

Littman disclosed that *Cryptococcus neoformans* has a requirement for thiamine, and the addition of yeast extract or the use of enriched media such as brain heart infusion agar (BHI) stimulates growth and capsule production. On BHI blood agar incubated at 37° C., the organism forms creamy, mucoid, opaque, raised circular colonies in 48 to 72 hours. Characteristic encapsulation of the cells may be observed microscopically.

Clinical materials should be cultured at both 20° C. and 37° C., for inability to grow at 37° C. rules out *Cryptococcus neoformans*. However, other cryptococci may grow at the latter temperature also. For 20° C. incubation, material should be plated onto SDA containing antibacterial antibiotics to suppress contaminants. *C. neoformans* is sensitive to cycloheximide, therefore, this antibiotic must not be incorporated in the media. Littman oxgall agar is a valuable primary isolation medium for 20° C. incubation. It limits growth of fast spreading saprophytic fungi and restricts bacterial growth. The fungus is relatively slow growing on Littman medium. In five to six days, the colonies are opaque with a bluish cast derived from the dye in the medium. They later become greyish tan, butyrous in consistency, and develop a smooth, slightly raised surface. Subculturing or continued incubation may be necessary to demonstrate encapsulation.

Most clinical materials from animals cannot be successfully cultured on enriched media at 37° C. because of fast overgrowth by contaminants. Colonies grown at 20° C. on the restrictive media described above, and which are suggestive of *Cryptococcus neoformans*, should be plated on BHI agar or BHI blood agar for incubation at 37° C. On the latter medium, *C. neoformans* appears within 48 to 72 hours as opaque, creamy, mucoid, raised circular colonies. Faster growth (24 to 36 hours) can be obtained on Littman liver-spleen glucose blood agar. Slide preparations made from either of these media show encapsulated budding yeastlike cells on microscopic examination.

Clinical specimens such as spinal fluid, milk, urine and blood, obtained aseptically, may yield pure growth of *Cryptococcus neoformans* when cultured at 37° C. on enriched media. Penicillin and streptomycin, or chloramphenicol is usually added to suppress bacterial contaminants.

Recently some specialized restrictive media have been developed which allow primary isolation of *Cryptococcus neoformans* from heavily contaminated environments such as soil, air and avian nests. These media will no doubt be utilized by some laboratories for primary isolations from contaminated clinical specimens. Staib discovered that among the species of the genus *Cryptococcus*, only *C. neoformans* assimilates the purine creatinine. He showed that *C. neoformans* selectively absorbs a pigment derived from *Guizotia abyssinica* seeds (nigerseed) also, thereby causing the colony to become brown.[33] Shields and Ajello[34] prepared a medium for selective isolation of *C. neoformans* which employed creatinine as a nitrogen source, diphenyl ($C_6H_5C_6H_5$) and chloramphenicol as mold and bacterial inhibitors, and nigerseed extract as a specific color marker.

Botard and Kelley[35] have modified Littman oxgall agar by adding an extract of *Guizotia abyssinica* seeds. They reported that the modified media retained the superior ability of the parent media to suppress bacteria and contaminating molds and that only *Cryptococcus neoformans* developed the distinctive brown color described by Staib.[33]

For laboratory identification of *Cryptococcus neoformans*, the two previously mentioned cultural characteristics must be demonstrated, i.e., ability to grow at 37° C., and production of a mucinous capsule. In addition, the following tests should be performed: urease test, nitrate and carbon assimilation tests, and/or pathogenicity test. The inability of the organism to produce a mycelium is a useful confirmatory test, and some workers have used an agglutination test for supporting confirmation.[36]

Optimum growth of *Cryptococcus neoformans* is attained at an incubation temperature near 29° C., and its upper limit of heat tolerance is 39° C. Abundant growth is obtained at 37° C., and this is an important identification criterion because a nonpathogenic species, *Cryptococcus diffluens* (*C. neoformans* var. *innocuous*), and most other usually harmless species are unable to grow at this temperature. Weak growth is sometimes obtained at 37° C. with *Cryptococcus laurentii* and *Cryptococcus luteolus*.

Formation of a thick mucinous capsule is characteristic of *Cryptococcus neoformans* when growing in tissue and under proper conditions in culture. As was previously stated, the finding of encapsulated yeastlike organisms in spinal fluid is prima facie evidence of cryptococcosis. This is true also when similar organisms are found in bovine milk when typical clinical signs are evident. It should be pointed out that many nonpathogenic *Cryptococcus* species produce capsules also.

The test for urease production is especially useful for differentiating *Cryptococcus* species from the yeastlike *Candida* species and from the true yeasts. The organism to be tested is streaked on the surface of agar slants of Christensen's Urea Medium and is incubated at 25° C. Development of a deep purple-red color throughout the medium in 18 to 48 hours constitutes a positive urease test. In common with *Cryptococcus neoformans*, the saprophytic cryptococci produce urease also. The true yeasts and most common species of the genus *Candida*, except *Candida krusei*, are urease-negative.

Nitrogen assimilation is a stable characteristic of yeasts and is useful as a means for genus and species differentiation. *Cryptococcus neoformans* cannot assimilate nitrogen, a characteristic it shares with the nonpathogenic species *Cryptococcus laurentii* and *Cryptococcus luteolus*. *Cryptococcus diffluens* and the other nonpathogenic members of the genus do assimilate nitrogen. Potassium nitrate is the sole source of nitrogen in both the agar plate and broth tests. Peptone and ammonium sulfate, respectively, serve as control substances. Both techniques are described in detail elsewhere.[14,37] The organism grows only if it is able to assimilate the nitrogen in the test medium.

Cryptococcus neoformans lacks the ability to produce gas from any known carbohydrate, although it does produce acids from sugar. On the other hand, saprophytic yeasts are ready fermenters and produce both acid and gas—thus providing a convenient means for differentiation. Carbohydrates which are fermented are also assimilated, but the converse is not always true.[14]

In the carbon assimilation test, the ability of an organism to utilize a specific single carbohydrate is tested in an otherwise carbon-free medium. Only the organisms capable of assimilating the carbohydrate being tested will grow on the medium. Littman describes an agar plate test which employs a carbohydrate-free basal medium which is seeded with the test organism. After incubation for a few hours to dry the agar surface the plate is marked into sectors on the glass bottom, and small quantities of dry carbohydrates are deposited on the surface in each sector. Dextrose serves as a control, since all yeasts assimilate this source of carbon. A similar test, in which 20-percent solutions of the test carbohydrate sources are placed on the plates in sterile antibiotic assay cylinders, has been recommended.[32] With either test, after 48 hours incubation at 25° C., visible growth appears around those carbohydrates which the organism is capable of assimilating. *Cryptococcus neoformans* assimilates arabinose, cellobiose, dextrose, dulcitol, galactose, raffinose, sucrose, and xylose; it does not assimilate lactose or melobiose.

Cryptococcus neoformans lacks the ability to form a true mycelium. This important identifying characteristic can be tested on chlamydospore agar or on cornmeal agar and is another means of differentiating *C. neoformans* from *Candida species* that regularly produce mycelium in such media.

Pathogenicity Tests

Cryptococcus neoformans is the only regularly pathogenic species of the genus *Cryptococcus*. Six-week-old white Swiss mice, intracerebrally inoculated with 0.02–0.03 ml. of a saline suspension of the organism, usually die in four days to two weeks. A few earlier and later deaths will occur. Prior to death, usually the mice first become listless, develop rough hair coats, a hydrocephalus-like bulging of the cranium and, terminally, marked signs of CNS disturbance (incoordination and/or circling). Those still alive after two weeks should be sacrificed. Remove top of skull, obtain brain material with platinum loop, and examine in India ink for the presence of encapsulated yeastlike cells.

Two nonpathogenic species of *Cryptococcus*, *C. laurentii* and *C. luteolus*, sometimes exhibit a mild degree of virulence when inoculated intraperitoneally into white Swiss mice. These species were previously mentioned as sometimes exhibiting weak growth on media at 37° C. also. Both of these species fail to assimilate nitrate. The problem of differentiating these and the other nonpathogenic cryptococci from *C. neoformans* may be unequivocally resolved with the intracerebral mouse inoculation test.

White Swiss mice succumb to intravenous injection of *Cryptococcus neoformans* via the tail vein in approximately two weeks. Following this method of inoculation, lesions may be found in the spleen, liver, lungs and brain.

Rats and guinea pigs are less susceptible than mice to experimental infection with *Cryptococcus neoformans*. Rabbits, due presumably to their high body temperature (39.5° C.), usually prove nonsusceptible to experimental injections.

Immunology

In comparison to other systemic mycotic disease agents, little is known about the immunology of *Cryptococcus neoformans*. The question of the occurrence of a benign form of cryptococcosis in man and animals has not been satisfactorily answered. Due partially to the absence of a sensitive and specific skin test antigen, the prevalence of the disease remains obscure. Although progress is being made, satisfactory and universally reliable serology test antigens for use as epidemiologic and diagnostic tools are not presently available.

Cryptococcus neoformans is notable for its ability to invade tissues without eliciting marked inflammatory responses. This phenomenon, due conceivably to the relative nonantigenicity of the capsular polysaccharides, may account for the inability of the host to develop detectable humoral antibodies in diagnostic titers. This hypothesis seems particularly applicable to infections of the meninges and bovine mammary gland. On the other hand, many workers believe that most infected individuals mount effective immunologic defenses and attain immunity. Some speculate that an immunologic defect (known in other mycotic diseases) is responsible for dissemination of *C. neoformans* from the initial infection site.

Preparation of satisfactory in vitro antigens has been influenced by the presence of the "protective" capsular material. For experimental study, some workers have employed strains with small capsules; others have enzymatically degraded the capsules of large capsule strains.[38]

Three antigenic types of *Cryptococcus neoformans*, A, B and C, all associated with capsular polysaccharide, have been known for several years. Specific agglutination, precipitation and capsular reactions have been obtained with immune rabbit serum. Recently, Wilson and associates[39] added another antigenic type (designated D) to those previously studied. Kaufman and Blumer[40] have reported the development and evaluation of agglutination and fluorescent antibody procedures for the identification of *C. neoformans*. Some problems of cross-reactivity with *Candida albicans* were alleviated in a subsequent study by Pidcoe and Kaufman.[41]

DIFFERENTIAL DIAGNOSIS

Cryptococcosis should be considered in cats and dogs with vague and nonspecific signs of CNS or respiratory disease, especially if accompanied by nasal discharges. Clinically, the disease in cats closely mimics the thoracic form of malignant lymphoma. In either disease, superficial node involvement may cause dysphagia and this may be the only sign observed by the owner. Malignant lymphoma merits differential consideration in dogs also. Canine cryptococcosis is sometimes manifested as a persistent otitis, as refractory oral and nasal lesions, and may simulate other respiratory mycotic infections.

Cryptococcosis of the bovine mammary gland must be differentiated from mastitis caused by some bacterial species, *Mycoplasma* species,[42] and *Nocardia* species. In addition to *Cryptococcus neoformans*, other yeastlike organisms occasionally cause bovine mastitis and may require identification. Members of the genera *Candida*, *Geotrichum* and *Trichosporon* have been incriminated as causes of mastitis. In contrast to the cryptococci, all produce a true mycelium under proper conditions. Members of the genus *Trichosporon* produce both blastospores and arthrospores. The genus *Geotrichum* contains only one species, *G. candidum* (formerly *Oospora lactis*). On direct examination of clinical materials or of young colonies, only yeastlike cells may be seen. After continued growth, a true mycelium forms which is composed of chains of rectangular arthrospores. For descriptions of the *Candida* species, see Chapter 5 on candidiasis.

Equine cryptococcosis almost invariably is seen as a respiratory ailment where obstructive growths are found in the nasal sinuses along with nasal discharges. Differential consideration should be given to phycomycosis and rhinosporidiosis. In histopathologic sections, the mature endospores of *Rhinosporidium seeberi* are covered with a mucicarminophilic matrix. However, the marked morphologic differences between *R. seeberi* and *Cryptococcus neoformans* should prevent confusion between them.

EPIDEMIOLOGY

The isolation of *Cryptococcus neoformans* from fruit juice by Sanfelice[4] in 1894 and the isolation from milk by Klein[7] in 1901 were probably due to contamination with dust containing the fungus. Ajello[25] has stated that soil is the ultimate source of all infections caused by *C. neoformans*. The fungus has been isolated from soil in many parts of the world, from milk, the surface of a peach, wasp nests, grass, bodies of insects, butter, tinned milk and the slime flux of the mesquite bush. Aged or "weathered" pigeon droppings in towers, cupolas, and similar roosting and nesting areas frequently contain the organism. Soil beneath such areas sometimes contains both *C. neoformans* and *Histoplasma capsulatum*. Even the surface of healthy human skin has been the source of an isolate of *C. neoformans*. Another source of the fungus in nature was recently disclosed in a report of its isolation from bat guano.[43]

Emmons[44] first discovered the presence of *Cryptococcus neoformans* in soil, and in a subsequent study he revealed a significant ecologic relationship between the fungus and pigeon droppings.[45] In another study Emmons[46] found that pigeon manure was particularly suitable as a medium for the fungus. Fifty-seven percent of one hundred eleven samples of old pigeon nests (composed almost entirely of excreta), yielded isolations of *C. neoformans*.

The discovery by Staib[33] that creatinine, a constituent of bird urine, is assimilated only by *Cryptococcus neoformans* among members of the genus *Cryptococcus* provided an explanation for the bird dung-*C. neoformans* association. It is known that the fungus exists in many habitats not obviously related to the presence of birds; it is postulated that cells from such areas, carried by wind currents to concentrations of creatinine-rich bird excrement, are deposited in a natural medium favoring their growth and multiplication. Avian habitats thus become the prime source of human and animal infection.[25]

Littman[14] has pointed out that spontaneous infections of birds have not been reported, possibly because they are protected by their high body temperature. However recently with his co-workers he successfully produced systemic infection in pigeons following intracerebral inoculation.[47] To date, no one has been able to infect birds systemically by any other inoculation route. Therefore, until spontaneous avian infections are proved, we must assume that the role of birds in the avian-*C. neoformans* relationship is indirect.

In their discussion of cryptococcosis in man, Littman and Zimmerman state that "the respiratory tract is considered to be the usual portal of entry of the organism since many patients with cryptococcal meningitis give a history of recent respiratory infection."[14] Pappagianis recently endorsed their view as follows: "Despite the

11

emphatic and classical association with meningitis or meningoencephalitis, there is increasing reason to believe on clinical grounds, too, that cryptococcosis is primarily a pulmonary infection."[48] Smith and associates[49] have provided some supportive evidence by demonstrating infection of mice with airborne *Cryptococcus neoformans.*

Mycotic diseases of animals vary, often greatly, in their manifestations in different species. Animal fungal infections, particularly in dogs, closely resemble their counterpart in man. However, similarities are not applicable as a general rule, and some signs exhibited by animals are rarely or never observed in human patients. Perhaps the most obvious example is cryptococcal bovine mastitis.

The above points are presented to introduce a debatable question. Are the lungs the primary focus for infections in animal cryptococcosis? The answer is obviously no in bovine mastitis. It seems reasonable, however, to question a primary pulmonary site in horses. Some persons will agree that nasal mucosa is a more likely site of primary infection in equine cases, for almost without exception, the lesions are confined to the nasal cavity and surrounding osseous structures. Several cases in dogs and cats with extensive pulmonary involvement and without obvious external lesions suggest the lungs as the primary infective focus. On the other hand, a significant number have prominent facial, nasal and aural lesions, and lung involvement in many of these cases has not been demonstrated. The final answer may await the results of experimental infections in the individual animal species.

Both man and animals become infected with *Cryptococcus neoformans* from exogenous sources in nature. There is no evidence of individual-to-individual or of animal-to-man transmission.

TREATMENT

See Chapter 7, treatment of systemic mycoses, pp. 102–103.

REFERENCES

 1. Freeman, W. J.: Torula Infection of the Central Nervous System. J. f. Psychol. u. Neurol., *43* (1931): 236.
 2. Busse, O.: Ueber Saccharomycosis Hominis. Virchow. Arch. Path. Anat., *140* (1895): 23–46.
 3. Buschke, A.: Ueber eine durch Coccidien Hervorgerufene Krankheit des Menschen. Deutsch. Med. Wschr., *21* (1895): 14.
 4. Sanfelice, F.: Contributo alla Morfologia e Biologia dei Blastomiceti. Ann. Igene Sper., *4* (1894): 463–495.
 5. Barron, C. N.: Cryptococcosis in Animals. J. Amer. Vet. Med. Ass., *127* (1955): 125–132.
 6. Vuillemin, P.: Les Blastomycetes Pathogenea. Rev. Gen. Sci. Pures Appl., *12* (1901): 732–751.
 7. Klein, E.: Pathogenic Microbes in Milk. J. Hyg., *1* (1901): 78–95.
 8. Weis, J. D.: Four Pathogenic Torulae (Blastomycetes). J. Med. Res. (New Series), *2* (1902): 280–311.
 9. Frothingham, L.: A Tumor-like Lesion in the Lung of a Horse Caused by a Blastomyces (Torula). J. Med. Res., *8* (1902): 31–43.
10. Verse, M.: Uber einen Fall von Generalisierter Blastomykose beim Menschen. Verh. Deutsch. Ges. Path., *17* (1914): 275–278.
11. Stoddard, J. L. and Cutler, E. C.: Torula Infection in Man. Monogr. Rockefeller Inst. Med. Res., *6* (1916): 1–98.
12. Emmons, C. W., Binford, C. H. and Utz, J. P.: *Medical Mycology.* 2nd edition, Philadelphia, Lea & Febiger, 1970.

13. Benham, R. W.: Cryptococci—Their Identification by Morphology and by Serology. J. Infect. Dis., *57* (1935): 255–274.
14. Littman, M. L. and Zimmerman, L. E.: *Cryptococcosis*. New York, Grune & Stratton, Inc., 1956.
15. Holzworth, J.: Cryptococcosis in a Cat. Cornell Vet., *42* (1952): 12–15.
16. Holzworth, J. and Coffin, D. L.: Cryptococcosis in a Cat: A Second Case. Cornell Vet., *43* (1953): 546–550.
17. Seibold, H. R., Roberts, C. S. and Jordan, E. M.: Cryptococcosis in a Dog. J. Amer. Vet. Med. Ass., *122* (1953): 213–215.
18. Wilson, J. W. and Plunkett, O. A.: *The Fungous Diseases of Man*. Berkeley, University of California Press, 1965.
19. Maddy, K. T.: Epidemiology and Ecology of Deep Mycoses of Man and Animals. Arch. Derm., *96* (1967): 409–417.
20. Pounden, W. D., Anderson, J. M. and Jaeger, R. F.: A Severe Mastitis Probelm Associated with *Cryptococcus Neoformans* in a Large Dairy Herd. Amer. J. Vet. Res., *13* (1952): 121–128.
21. Innes, J. R. M., Seibold, H. R. and Arentzen, W. P.: The Pathology of Bovine Mastitis Caused by *Cryptococcus Neoformans*. Amer. J. Vet. Res., *13* (1952): 469–475.
22. Emmons, C. W.: *Cryptococcus Neoformans* Strains from a Severe Outbreak of Bovine Mastitis. Mycopathologia, *6* (1952): 231–234.
23. Simon, J., Nichols, R. E. and Morse, E. V.: An Outbreak of Bovine Cryptococcosis. J. Amer. Vet. Med. Ass., *122* (1953): 31–35.
24. Ajello, L.: Occurrence of *Cryptococcus Neoformans* in Soils. Amer. J. Hyg., *67* (1958): 72–77.
25. Ajello, L.: Comparative Ecology of Respiratory Mycotic Disease Agents. Bact. Rev., *31* (1967): 6–24.
26. Marcato, P. S.: A Case of Hodgkin's Disease Associated with Cryptococcosis in a Dog. J. Small Anim. Pract., *7* (1966): 649–651.
27. Weidman, F. O., in discussion of Wile, U. J.: Cutaneous Torulosis. Arch. Dermat. Syph., *31* (1935): 58–66.
28. Okoshi, S. and Hasegawa, A.: Cryptococcosis in a Cat. Jap. J. Vet. Sci., *30* (1968): 39–42.
29. Wagner, J. L., James, R. P. and Krigman, M. R.: *Cryptococcus Neoformans* Infection in a Dog. J. Amer. Vet. Med. Ass., *153* (1968): 945–949.
30. Smith, H. A., Jones, T. C. and Hunt, R. D.: *Veterinary Pathology*. 4th edition, Philadelphia, Lea & Febiger, 1972.
31. Carter, H. S. and Young, J. L.: Note on the Isolation of *Cryptococcus Neoformans* from a Sample of Milk. J. Path. Bact., *62* (1950): 271–273.
32. Ajello, L., Georg, L. K., Kaplan, W. and Kaufman, L.: *Laboratory Manual for Medical Mycology*. Washington, U. S. Govt. Printing Office, 1963.
33. Staib, F.: New Concepts in the Occurrence and Identification of *Cryptococcus Neoformans*. Mycopathologia, *19* (1963): 143–145.
34. Shields, A. B. and Ajello, L.: Medium for Selective Isolation of *Cryptococcus neoformans*. Science, *151* (1966): 208–209.
35. Botard, R. W. and Kelley, D. C.: Modified Littman Oxgall Agar to Isolate *Cryptococcus neoformans*. Appl. Microbiol., *16* (1968): 689–690.
36. Sotgin, G., Mazzoni, A., Mantovani, A., Ajello, L. and Palmer, J.: Survey of Soils for Human Pathogenic Fungi from the Eimilia-Romagna Region of Italy. II. Isolation of *Allescheria boydii*, *Cryptococcus neoformans* and *Histoplasma capsulatum*. Amer. J. Epidemiol., *83* (1966): 329–337.
37. *Basic Techniques and Newer Concepts in Clinical Diagnostic Medical Mycology*. St. Louis, Catholic Hospital Association, 1960.
38. Kong, Y. M. and Levine, H. B.: Experimentally Induced Immunity in the Mycoses. Bact. Rev., *31* (1967): 35–53.
39. Wilson, D. E., Bennett, J. E. and Bailey, J. W.: Serologic Grouping of *Cryptococcus neoformans*. Proc. Soc. Exp. Biol. Med., *127* (1968): 820–823.

40. Kaufman, L. and Blumer, S.: Development and Evaluation of Agglutination and Fluorescent Antibody Procedures for the Identification of *Cryptococcus neoformans.* Sabouraudia, *4* (1965): 57–64.

41. Pidcoe, V. and Kaufman, L.: Fluorescent-Antibody Reagent for the Identification of *Cryptococcus neoformans.* Appl. Microbiol., *16* (1968): 271–275.

42. Jasper, D. E.: Mycoplasmas: Their Role in Bovine Disease. J. Amer. Vet. Med. Ass., *151* (1967): 1650–1655.

43. Ajello, L., Hosty, T. S. and Palmer, J.: Bat Histoplasmosis in Alabama. Amer. J. Trop. Med., *16* (1967): 329–331.

44. Emmons, C. W.: Isolation of *Cryptococcosis neoformans* from Soil. J. Bact., *62* (1951): 685–690.

45. Emmons, C. W.: Saprophytic Sources of *Cryptococcus neoformans* Associated with Pigeon (*Columba livia*). Amer. J. Hyg., *62* (1955): 227–232.

46. Emmons, C. W.: Natural Occurrence of Opportunistic Fungi. J. Lab. Invest., *11* (1962): 1026–1032.

47. Littman, M. L., Borok, R. and Dalton, J. G.: Experimental Avian Cryptococcosis. Amer. J. Epidemiology, *82* (1965): 197–207.

48. Pappagianis, D.: Epidemiological Aspects of Respiratory Mycotic Infections. Bact. Rev., *31* (1967): 25–34.

49. Smith, C. D., Ritter, R., Larsh, H. W. and Furcolow, M. L.: Infection of White Swiss Mice with Airborne *Cryptococcus neoformans.* J. Bact., *87* (1964): 1364–1368.

Part IV
THE ACTINOMYCETOSES

CHAPTER **11** | Actinomycosis

Actinomycosis is a chronic infectious disease of animals and man caused by micro-aerophilic to anaerobic species of the genus *Actinomyces*. The usual etiologic agents in cattle and man are *Actinomyces bovis* and *Actinomyces israelii*, respectively. Bovine infections characteristically involve the mandible, less often the maxilla, causing a suppurative or proliferative osteitis commonly called "lumpy jaw." Other than in cattle and possibly in swine and dogs, animal infections are rare.

HISTORY, GEOGRAPHIC DISTRIBUTION AND PREVALENCE

Bollinger in a talk in 1876 was the first to describe granules in the suppurative exudate from lesions of cattle having the disease commonly known to veterinarians as "lumpy jaw." In a paper published in 1877,[1] Bollinger indicated that material from such bovine lesions had been sent to the botanist Harz for study, and that Harz[2] gave the name *Actinomyces bovis* (literally, "ray-fungus of the cow") to the filamentous organisms that were observed microscopically in the granules. The disease was called actinomycosis. The organism had not been isolated in culture from bovine clinical material.

A similar disease of the cervico-facial areas of human beings was recognized at about this same time. Because of the similarity to the disease of cattle described by Bollinger and Harz, it was called actinomycosis also. A filamentous organism was isolated in pure culture and characterized from human clinical material by Wolff and Israel[3] in 1891. This organism was named *Streptothrix israelii* by Kruse in 1896 but was later placed in the genus *Actinomyces* by Lachner-Sandoval in 1896 as *Actinomyces israelii*.

For many years it was believed that *Actinomyces bovis* and *A. israelii* were the same organism, and the name *A. bovis* was used by many workers for the etiologic agent of both animal and human actinomycosis since this name had priority.

In 1940, however, Erickson in Scotland carried out a careful comparative study of bovine and human isolates and presented evidence that these were not the same species. Although the two organisms appeared the same in the granules, *i.e.*, as highly filamentous, branched forms, in culture the cattle isolates were largely diphtheroidal in form and produced smooth colonies; while human isolates remained highly filamentous and produced rough colonies. Besides these morphologic differences, she pointed out differences in biochemical reactions as well as serologic differences.[5]

More recent studies in the United States confirm the work of Erickson (Thompson,[6] 1950; Pine, Howell and Watson,[7] 1960; Lambert, Brown and Georg,[20] 1967), and it is now accepted that these are indeed two distinct species. The name *Actinomyces bovis* is reserved for the species usually isolated from bovine infections and *A. israelii* for the species usually isolated from human infections.

These two species are not, however, host specific as *Actinomyces israelii* has been isolated at least twice from bovine infections. To our knowledge, however, *A. bovis* has not been isolated from human material (Pine, Howell and Watson,[7] Georg, Robertstad and Brinkman[11]).

Several concepts of actinomycosis in animals have either been proven erroneous or are highly questionable, yet some tend to persist in reports and textbooks. A bulletin published in 1935 stated, "This fungus finds very favorable conditions outside the animal body for its growth."[8] At present it is a disputed point whether or not *Actinomyces bovis* has a natural habitat outside the animal body. It has not yet been isolated from soil or plants.[9]

Several bacterial and fungal pathogens produce lesions, and in some cases exudates, that are quite similar to those of actinomycosis. No doubt many early animal cases reported as actinomycosis were caused by *Nocardia* spp. or the bacterial pathogens *Actinobacillus lignieresii*, *Staphylococcus aureus* and *Corynebacterium* spp. A case in point is the often cited report of an etiologic role of *Actinomyces bovis* in "fistulous withers" and "poll evil" of horses. Mycologists have questioned the efficacy of *A. bovis* in these equine maladies for several years. Competent workers have studied the biochemical reactions of the questioned isolates and concluded that they were not actinomycetes.[7] Another report of equine actinomycosis involving a mandibular lymph node lacked sufficient data for precise identification of the causal agent.[10]

The question of a causal role of *Actinomyces bovis* in actinomycosis of dogs, cats, swine, other domestic and some wild animals is unanswered. Many isolates from these animals were not completely studied and described. No doubt many were *Actinomyces* spp., but available data does not allow precise species identification. In respect to the many authors involved, it must be pointed out that only in very recent years has knowledge accumulated which permits positive identification of the pathogenic *Actinomyces* spp. To date, using the criteria of thorough biochemical and serologic study, researchers have identified *A. bovis* only from bovine cases.

An obvious need exists for thorough studies of isolates from other animal species, particularly swine. Actinomycotic infection of the porcine mammary gland is generally considered to occur frequently. Many of these infections are possibly staphylococcic "botryomycosis," nocardiosis or actinobacillosis. All of these infections may cause granulomatous or suppurative lesions and may produce granules with clubbing as in true actinomycosis. Studies are needed to determine the relative incidence of true actinomycosis and to clarify the identity of the causal organism. Grasser's reports from Germany of the isolation of *Actinomyces israelii* and another species he designated *Actinomyces suis* from swine mammary infections need confirmation.[12,13]

Facultative or anaerobic diphtheroids sometimes cause suppurative or granulo-

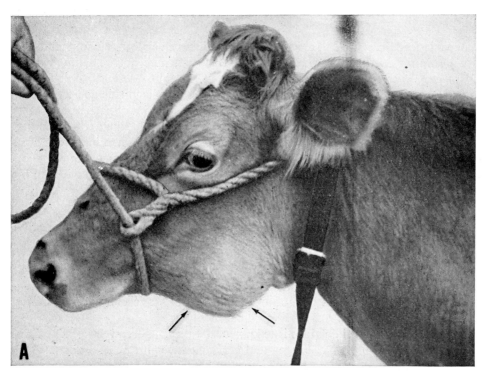

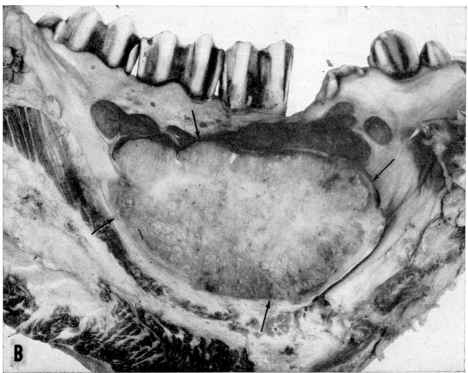

Fig. 11–1. Actinomycosis. **A.** Lesions in mandible of a Guernsey cow. Case from clinic of College of Veterinary Medicine, Iowa State College. **B.** Gross specimen from mandible of a similar case. AFIP 18198. Contributor: Major Lytle, V.C. (Smith, Jones and Hunt, Veterinary Pathology, courtesy of Lea & Febiger)

matous lesions in animals resembling true actinomycosis but without clubbing granules in the exudates, a usual but not consistent feature of true actinomycosis. *Corynebacterium pyogenes* and *C. acnes* are found in animal lesions, sometimes in association with actinomycetes; they cause both clinical diagnostic and laboratory identification problems. *C. acnes* is not described in veterinary bacteriology texts and a study of its animal associations would be a welcome addition to the literature.

Actinomycosis of cattle and man are similar clinically. Human infections most commonly affect the cervico-facial region, however, abdominal and thoracic infections are seen frequently. Infection often follows tooth extraction and injury to the mouth and jaw. Human infections are considered to be endogenous, as *Actinomyces israelii* is a common commensal of the mouth with the tonsilar crypts and carious teeth serving as reservoirs.

Bovine actinomycosis is usually cervico-facial with most infections involving the mandible or subcutaneous tissues of the lower jaw. Although *Actinomyces bovis* infections can extend by slow progression into contiguous tissues or rarely by the bloodstream, generalized infections are apparently rare. A culturally and serologically proven case of bovine pulmonary actinomycosis has recently been described by Biever and colleagues.[14]

The source of bovine infections is unknown, but they apparently are endogenous also. *Actinomyces bovis* has oxygen and enrichment requirements which make it doubtful that the organism can survive for long in nature.

Bovine actinomycosis occurs throughout the world wherever cattle are kept. In the United States the infection apparently is more prevalent in the central and northern states where roughages are fed in the winter season. The incidence appears to be higher where bearded grain straw and ensilage are fed. These feeds have a potential for injuring and penetrating the oral mucosa.

The writer has observed herds with a high incidence of actinomycosis in which most of the cattle between eighteen months and four years of age were infected. Shedding of deciduous and eruption of permanent teeth in this age group with companion oral inflammatory lesions was considered to be a contributing factor.

CLINICAL SIGNS AND PATHOLOGY

Often bovine actinomycosis is observed first as a circumscribed, hard, immovable protuberance of the mandible or maxilla. Usually the lesion is located in dorso-ventral alignment with the molar teeth. The infection destroys bone and simultaneously stimulates bony growth thereby causing a proliferative osteitis which is commonly called "lumpy jaw." In some cases there is extensive production of connective tissue in the adjacent subcutaneous tissues, varying from soft to hard, depending upon the predominance of suppurative or granulomatous reactions. Occasionally there is extensive enlargement in the intramandibular space or turbinate sinuses with little external swelling. These may impair mastication or breathing.

In the more typical cases, large granulomatous swellings appear on the surface of the jaw followed by the appearance of sinus tracts. These discharge a thick, mucoid, yellowish purulent exudate which may or may not contain granules with clubbing. If present, the granules are firm and white to yellowish in color, hence the designation "sulfur granules." Occasionally a sinus will heal, forming a depressed, indurated scar with the skin firmly adherent to the bone. Rarely a sinus tract will open to the oral cavity, and the teeth may become malaligned and loosened.

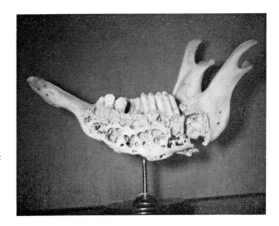

Fig. 11–2. Museum specimen of bovine mandible showing bone destruction and proliferation resulting from *A. bovis* infection.

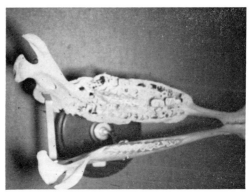

Fig. 11–3. Dorsal view of mandible in Fig. 11–2.

Some lesions develop rapidly, attaining a diameter of several inches in a period of weeks. However, most develop over a period of months. Some, particularly treated cases, appear to have periodic remissions of growth. The general health of the affected animal remains good as long as mastication is not impaired and individuals have remained productive for several years.

Grossly, the cut surface of the lesion may appear shining white due to the firm and dense consistency of the fibrous tissue. Small abscesses may be seen within the granulation, and these often contain "sulfur granules" (colonies of the organism). The abscesses often coalesce with subsequent development of sinus tracts which may invade adjacent bone. The infected bone undergoes rarefaction necrosis with concurrent proliferative regeneration. The organism does not spread via the lymphatic vessels and does not invade local nodes as is common with *Actinobacillus lignieresii* infections.

Microscopically, the individual suppurative lesions are found within a zone of neutrophils which are surrounded by an outer area of large mononuclear (epithelioid) cells with abundant, often foamy, cytoplasm. Giant cells of the Langhans type and lymphocytes are occasionally found in this region. The dense, moderately vascular connective tissue that separates the many abscesses from one another usually encapsulates the entire lesion.[15]

In fixed histopathologic sections the granules of actinomycosis contain grampositive, non-acid-fast, branched filaments in the interior when stained by the

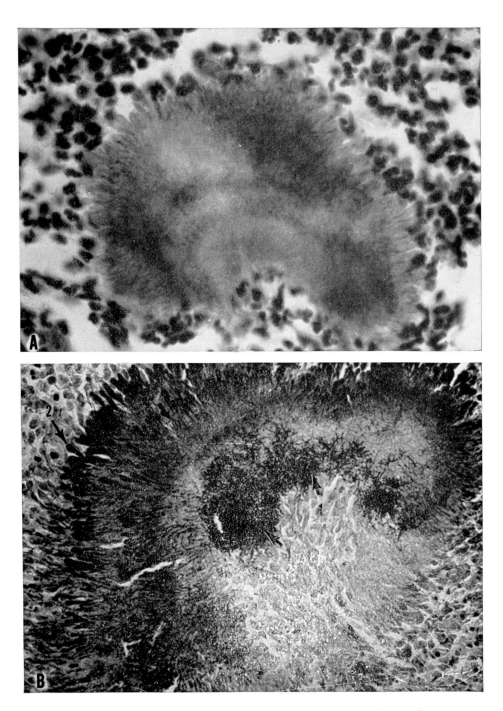

Fig. 11–4. Actinomycosis. **A.** Colony of *Actinomyces bovis* ($\times$ 500), in a tissue section stained with hematoxylin and eosin. AFIP 18198. Contributor: Major Lytle, V.C. **B.** A similar colony of *Actinomyces bovis* ($\times$ 500) in a tissue section stained by Gram's method. Note tangled, branching, Gram-positive organisms in the center (1) surrounded by zones of radiating club-shaped structure (2). AFIP 129816. Contributor: Dr. H. R. Seibold. (Smith, Jones and Hunt, Veterinary Pathology, courtesy of Lea & Febiger)

Brown and Brenn modification of the Gram stain and the Fite-Faraco acid-fast stain modified for *Nocardia* spp.[16] With more commonly used H and E or PAS stains, the granules are stained but the enclosed filamentous organisms are not.

LABORATORY DIAGNOSIS

Because of the probability of bacterial contamination of exudative material from draining sinuses, the collection site first should be thoroughly cleaned and disinfected. Preferably, pus should be aspirated from unopened lesions into a sterile syringe. Usually the abscess will be discharging, and exudates should be obtained either by aspiration or curettement. If sterile gauze is lightly packed into the sinus for a time, exudative material containing characteristic "sulfur granules" may adhere to it upon removal.

If granules are present, they may be grossly visible in the exudate. They may be trapped in the pus, and vigorous shaking in sterile saline within a closed container will usually free them and they will settle to the bottom. The granules vary from barely visible specks to 5 mm in diameter, are firm to hard and are white to yellow in color.

Direct Microscopic Examination

Granules should be placed in a drop of water, gently pressed under a coverslip and examined under low power in reduced light for an irregular, clubbed surface. Clubbing may not be observed always. Furthermore, granules with clubs may occur in other infections. Their diagnostic significance has been overestimated.[9] It is important to observe the preparation under oil immersion for delicate filaments which may be present within the granules and extend into the clubs.

Several smears of crushed granules should be prepared for Gram and acid-fast stains (Kinyoun's acid-fast cold stain using one-percent H_2SO_4 for decolorization).

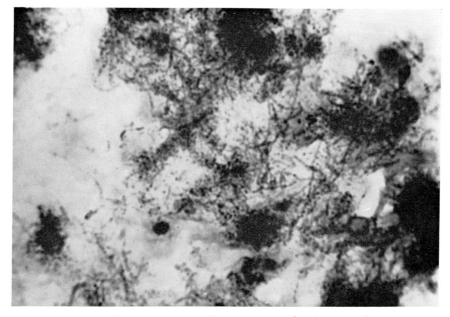

Fig. 11–5. Gram stain of *Actinomyces bovis* in exudate.

Examine stained smears under oil immersion for thin, non-acid-fast filaments which may show branching. Pleomorphic, sometimes branched forms of bacillary size may predominate or be the only forms observed. Stains of old colonies which have undergone degenerative changes may stain poorly or appear as gram-negative, rod-shaped bacteria.

If granules are not found, make smears for staining of pus, blood flecks, tissue fragments or centrifuged washings from gauze tampons.

Culture

The *Actinomyces* spp. are microaerophilic to anaerobic. Usually *A. bovis* is more aerotolerant than *A. israelii*. However, anaerobic methods should be used for isolation. Culture of granules affords the best chance for a successful isolation. Granules should be crushed after thorough washing in sterile saline. Other materials should be washed several times also, then centrifuged to obtain sediment for inoculation. Both liquid and solid media should be used for isolation attempts.

Enriched liquid thioglycollate broth, freshly boiled, and fresh Brain Heart Infusion (BHI) agar are recommended. Some workers include blood agar and casitone-starch medium for isolation. All media should have a pH between 6.8 and 7.2 and cultures should be incubated under anaerobic conditions at 37° C. If anaerobe jars without catalyst are used, an atmosphere of 95-percent N_2 and 5-percent CO_2 is recommended. Culture transfers to tubed media may be incubated in anaerobe jars or under "anaerobe seals" (pyrogallic acid + Na_2CO_3).

On agar plates the colonies of *Actinomyces bovis* are characteristically smooth whereas those of *A. israelii* usually are rough. This morphologic characteristic results from the quantity of filamentation produced. Variations occur between isolates and sometimes in subculture, but colony morphology generally is uniform to species. Occasionally, rough types of *A. bovis* and smooth types of *A. israelii* are isolated. The student is cautioned that the diptheroids, *Corynebacterium pyogenes* and *C. acnes*, may resemble the smooth type of *Actinomyces* spp. on agar.

Agar colonies of *Actinomyces bovis* usually are tiny, shining, "dew-droplike," convex and entire. They are not hemolytic on blood agar. Older colonies are low convex, entire, off-white in color and soft in consistency. In thioglycollate broth, *A. bovis* produces a soft, diffuse growth.

Agar colonies of *Actinomyces israelii* develop more slowly than those of *A. bovis*. Grossly, one- to two-day colonies are barely visible. Under 10× magnification they appear as delicately branched filaments ("spider colonies"). Older colonies (seven to ten days) develop a heaped, rough surface ("molar tooth colony"). They are firm in consistency and partially embedded in the agar. They are not hemolytic on blood agar. Discrete, granular or "bread crumb" colonies are formed in thioglycollate broth which remains clear.

Biochemical tests for identification should include a determination of catalase production. *Corynebacterium acnes* is catalase-positive which differentiates it from the catalase-negative *Actinomyces* spp. Other useful tests include hemolysis, reaction in milk, nitrate reduction, gelatin liquefaction, starch hydrolysis and sugar fermentations.

Smith and Holdeman[17] state that a strain of nonmotile, anaerobic, non-sporing, gram-positive rods, showing slight branching, not producing catalase, not liquefying gelatin, not producing hemolysis on blood agar, not fermenting mannose, not re-

TABLE 11–1. Biochemical Characteristics of Actinomyces and
Corynebacterium Species*

	A. bovis	A. israelii	C. pyogenes	C. acnes**
Hemolysis	—	—	+	—
Nitrate red	—(v)	+(+)	—	+
Catalase production	—	—	—	+
Gelatin liquefaction	—	—(v)	+	+
			(1–2 wks.)	
Indol	—	—	—	v
Starch hydrolysis	+	—(v)	+	—
Litmus milk	acid	— or acid	coag., 48 hrs; acid + digestion, late. soft coag.	

(v) = rarely variable from reaction shown.

Fermentation (acid, 7 days)				
dextrose	+	+	+	+
maltose	v	+	+	—
lactose	+	+	+	—
sucrose	+	+	+	—
mannitol	v	v	—	v
galactose	v	v	+	v
salicin	v	+	—	—
arabinose	v	v	—	—
fructose	+	+	+	+
xylose	v	+	+	—
starch	+	—	+	—
dextrin	+	+	+	—
glycerol	v	—	v	+

+ = acid; v = variable; — = no acid.
* Modified from Ajello, L. et al., CDC Laboratory Manual for Medical Mycology, Washington, U.S. Dept. of Health, Education and Welfare, Public Health Service.
** Moss, et al., J. Bact., 94 (167): 1300–1305.

ducing nitrate, but hydrolyzing starch may be tentatively identified as *Actinomyces bovis.*

A strain with gram-positive branching rods, non-sporing, obligately anaerobic, not producing catalase, not liquefying gelatin, not producing hemolysis, but reducing nitrate and fermenting mannose but not mannitol may be tentatively identified as *Actinomyces israelii.*[17]

Pathogenicity Tests

Animal inoculations are of limited value in the identification of *Actinomyces* spp. and are not routinely done. A small percentage of hamsters will develop lesions following intraperitoneal inoculation, and these may be used as a source of material for classroom study.

mmunology

A dependable test for the detection of antibodies in animal serum is not available. Specific antibodies can be experimentally produced in laboratory animals, and these have been successfully used to differentiate *Actinomyces* spp. by agar gel precipitin and fluorescent antibody tests.[18,19,20] Reagent antigens and antiserums are not generally available at present.

DIFFERENTIAL DIAGNOSIS

Actinomycosis must be differentiated from nocardiosis, actinobacillosis, staphylococcic "botryomycosis," and other bacterial infections, notably those caused by *Corynebacterium* spp.

EPIDEMIOLOGY

The pathogenic *Actinomyces* spp. have never been found other than in intimate relationships to man and animals. It is established that *A. israelii* is a common commensal in the mouth of humans and that it has the ability to invade injured oral tissues. It seems safe to assume that *A. bovis* is endogenous to cattle as a commensal also and that trauma to the oral mucosa is important to its attaining virulence. It is unknown whether *A. bovis* is present in the mouth of other animal species. Although the organism has been reported in swine, the identification was not adequate by present standards.

Animal-to-animal transmission of actinomycosis apparently does not occur. Transfer of the organism from cow to calf immediately following parturition during licking and cleanup of the calf seems a logical assumption.

There is no evidence of animal-to-man transmission, neither are there any well-authenticated records of *Actinomyces bovis* infection in humans.

TREATMENT

The prognosis in actinomycosis therapy varies from good to poor depending upon the duration, extent and location of the lesion, and especially upon the extent of bone involvement. Early lesions in soft tissue and those with minimal bone invasion respond most favorably. Surgical drainage and curettement are important. Packing of cavities and tracts with Lugol's iodine or escharotic agents is beneficial also.

Actinomyces bovis is sensitive to iodides and penicillin. However, the infective agent is often "protected" by virtue of its presence deep in sinus tracts and bone or surrounded by exudates and granulation tissue. Therefore, prolonged therapy is indicated. Potassium iodide orally (one-eighth to one-fourth ounce daily), or sodium iodide intravenously (one-half to one ounce in 250–500 ml. diluent once or twice weekly), may be continued until signs of iodism appear. After a few weeks' interval, the treatment may be repeated if necessary. Concurrent use of penicillin may be helpful.

Because of the difficulty in clinically differentiating actinomycosis from actinobacillosis, and the probability of the gram-negative agent of actinobacillosis being sensitive to streptomycin, some veterinarians routinely supplement iodide therapy with penicillin and streptomycin in combination. Some clinicians inject streptomycin around the periphery of the granulomatous and bony protuberances in the hope of arresting and reducing the enlargement. This procedure has been disappointing to the author; in fact, it sometimes apparently has stimulated enlargement of the lesion. Chemotherapy should not be expected to reduce exostosis but to arrest it only. Exacerbation may occur months after bony proliferation has been seemingly arrested completely. Retreatment may be successful, and individuals have remained productive and profitable for months or years.

X-irradiation has been used as supplemental therapy in bovine actinomycosis with variable results. Repeated treatments are required and care must be taken to prevent overexposure and necrosis.

Bovine actinomycosis has been successfully treated with isoniazid (Nydrazid*) given in the feed at a dosage of 20 mg./kg. daily for 100 days.[21] No undesirable side effects were noted. Suppuration stopped and bony growth was arrested in 14 cows treated with 4 to 5 Gm. on the feed once daily for two to three weeks.[22]

REFERENCES

1. Bollinger, O: Ueber eine neue Pilzkrankheit bein Rinde. Centralbl. f.d. med. Wissensch., *15* (1877): 481–485.
2. Harz, C. O.: *Actinomyces bovis*, ein neuer Schimmel in den Geweben des Rindes. Deutsch. Z. Tiermed., *5* (1879): 123–140.
3. Wolff, M. and Israel, J.: Ueber Reincultur des Actinomyces und seine Uebertragbarkeit auf Thiere. Virchow. Arch. Path. Anat., *128* (1891): 11–59.
4. Francis, M.: Lump Jaw of Cattle. In Texas Agri. Expt. Station Bulletin No. 30 (1894): 448–449.
5. Erickson, D.: Pathogenic Anaerobic Microorganisms of the Actinomyces Group. Med. Res. Council (Brit.) Spec. Rep. Ser. No. 240 (1940): 1–63.
6. Thompson, L.: Isolation and Comparison of Actinomyces from Human and Bovine Infections. Proc. Mayo Clin., *25* (1950): 81–96.
7. Pine, L., Howell, A., Jr. and Watson, S. J.: Studies of the Morphological, Physiological and Biochemical Characters of *Actinomyces bovis*. J. Gen. Microbiol., *23* (1960): 403–424.
8. Connaway, J. W. and Uren, A. W.: Actinomycosis in Cattle. Univ. of Mo., Agri. Expt. Station Bulletin No. *357* (1935): 1–16.
9. Ajello, L., Georg, L. K., Kaplan, W. and Kaufman L.: *Laboratory Manual for Medical Mycology*. Washington, U. S. Gov't Printing Office, 1963.
10. Burns, R. H. G. and Simmons, G. C.: A Case of Actinomycotic Infection in a Horse. Aust. Vet. J. (1952): 34–35.
11. Georg, L. K., Robertstad, G. W. and Brinkman, S. A.: Identification of Species of Actinomyces. J. Bact., *88* (1964): 477–490.
12. Grasser, R.: Mikroaerophile Actinomyceten aus Gesaugeaktinomykosen des Schweines. Zbl. Bakt. [Orig.], *184* (1962): 478–492.
13. Grasser, R.: Untersuchungen uber Fermentative und Serologische Eigenschaften Mikroaerophiler-Actinomyceten. Zbl. Bakt. [Orig.], *188* (1963): 251–263.
14. Biever, L. J., Robertstad, G. W., Van Steenbergh, K., Scheetz, E. E. and Kennedy, G. F.: Actinomycosis in a Bovine Lung. Amer. J. Vet. Res., *30* (1969): 1063–1066.
15. Smith, H. A., Jones, T. C. and Hunt, R. D.: *Veterinary Pathology*. 4th edition, Philadelphia, Lea & Febiger, 1972.
16. Emmons, C. W., Binford, C. H. and Utz, J. P.: *Medical Mycology*. 2nd edition, Philadelphia, Lea & Febiger, 1970.
17. Smith, L. D. and Holdeman, L. V.: *The Pathogenic Anaerobic Bacteria*. Springfield, Charles C Thomas, 1968.
18. Blank, C. and Georg, L. K.: The Use of Fluorescent Antibody Methods for the Detection and Identification of *Actinomyces* Species in Clinical Material. J. Lab. Clin. Med., *71* (1968): 283–293.
19. Slack, J. and Gerenscer, M. A.: Revision of Serological Groupings of *Actinomyces*. J. Bact., *91* (1966): 2107.

* E. R. Squibb & Sons, New York, New York.

20. Lambert, F. W., Jr., Brown, J. M. and Georg, L. K.: Identification of *Actinomyces Israeli* and *A. Naeslundii* by Fluorescent-Antibody and Agar Gel Diffusion Techniques. J. Bact., *94* (1967): 1287–1295.
21. Ansbacher, S.: Treatment of Actinomycosis with Isoniazid. Vet. Med., *49* (1954): 357–358.
22. Brodie, B. and Manning, J. P.: Isoniazid Treatment of Actinomycosis. Mod. Vet. Practice, No. 11, *48* (1967): 70–71.

CHAPTER 12 | Nocardiosis

Nocardiosis is an acute or chronic suppurative or granulomatous disease of various animals and man caused by species of *Nocardia*, principally *Nocardia asteroides*. The disease may be systemic with primary pulmonary involvement followed by metastasis to other organs and lymph nodes. Localized and mycetoma type infections may result from injuries. Bovine mammary infections may cause serious economic loss.

HISTORY, GEOGRAPHIC DISTRIBUTION AND PREVALENCE

The first recorded case of nocardiosis was reported from cattle with farcy ("farcin de boeuf") on the island of Guadeloupe in the French West Indies by Nocard in 1888.[1] The aerobic actinomycete he isolated was accorded the binominal *Nocardia farcinica* by Trevisan in 1889. Although this name has priority, recent studies by Gordon and Mihm[2] of isolates in type-culture collections have apparently established that Nocard's original isolation was the species now recognized as *Nocardia asteroides*. They stated that although the name *Nocardia farcinica* has priority, replacement of the well-established and widely accepted name *Nocardia asteroides* by one which has nearly disappeared from culture collections and current literature does not serve the principle of the fixity of names.

Eppinger,[3] in 1891, isolated the organism now designated *Nocardia asteroides* from a brain abscess of a man who died of a generalized disease which resembled tuberculosis. He erroneously placed his isolate in the genus *Cladothrix*. It was changed to the genus *Nocardia* by Blanchard in 1895.[4]

The early literature which followed the original reports of Nocard and Eppinger does not clearly differentiate between nocardiosis and actinomycosis, and there was a great deal of confusion associated with identification, classification and nomenclature. The validity of many of the reports is impossible to establish. Many of the isolates were not adequately studied in culture, and some reports were based on studies of tissues only without the support of cultures. Careful study of some of the reports of nocardiosis which contain cultural data reveals that some of the isolates were other actinomycetes, and the diagnosis of nocardiosis was erroneous.

171

In common with many of the other pathogenic fungi, a conflicting synonymy has developed: *Cladothrix asteroides, Streptothrix eppingerii, Streptothrix carnea, Actinomyces gypsoides, Proactinomyces asteroides* and others. Gordon and Mihm[5] identified 79 strains of *Nocardia asteroides* received from individual donors and culture collections. When received, only 43 of the 79 strains were labeled *N. asteroides* or its varieties; 21 were submitted as 17 other species, and 15 merely as *Nocardia, Actinomyces* or *Streptomyces species.*

The occurrence of nocardiosis is reported in several different animal species in the early literature, but questionable cases materially reduce the different species incidence. For example, there are several references to the disease in horses, but none of them can be authenticated.

A significant number of early reports however, have been accepted as authentic.[6] Infection of the dog with *Nocardia asteroides* was first reported by Balozet and Pernot[7] in 1936. Ginsberg and Little[8] isolated this fungus from a dog in 1948. Their report was titled "Actinomycosis in Dogs" and this illustrates some of the nomenclature confusion in early literature. The genus *Nocardia* is in the family *Actinomycetaceae*, and early workers sometimes designated as actinomycosis diseases caused by *Nocardia* spp. Actinomycosis should be reserved for disease caused by members of the genus *Actinomyces.*

Soon after the report of Ginsberg and Little, the problems with classification and nomenclature were greatly diminished, and valid reports appeared with increasing frequency. Bohl and associates[9] first reported *Nocardia asteroides* infection in the dog in the United States in 1953. Other cases were reviewed by Maddy and co-workers[10] in 1955 when they reported on the eighth case definitely diagnosed as caused by *N. asteroides.* They stated that prior to their report, a literature review revealed that authenticated cases of *N. asteroides* infection had been found only in man and dogs.

There has been a marked increase in the reported cases in dogs and in other animal species, particularly cattle, in recent years. No doubt much of the increase can be attributed to improved diagnostic techniques, but accumulating evidence supports the contention that the incidence of nocardiosis is increasing. The hypothesis that the increase may be due in part to the widespread and sometimes indiscriminate use of antibiotic and adrenocortical steroid drugs seems fully acceptable.

Nocardia brasiliensis and *Nocardia caviae* have become established as etiologic agents of nocardiosis in animals and man also. Recent reports indicate that *N. brasiliensis* has a wider geographic distribution and greater prevalence and importance than has been determined previously.[11] *N. caviae* may cause rapidly fatal systemic infections in dogs[12,13] and this organism has been isolated from milk in bovine mastitis.[30]

Systemic feline nocardiosis from which *Nocardia asteroides* was isolated has been described by Langham and colleagues.[14] Ajello and partners[11] have reported the isolation of *N. brasiliensis* from a cat, the first authenticated lower animal infection due to this agent. They reviewed its prevalence and geographic distribution. This organism had previously been reported in error as the causal agent of bovine mastitis in Canada; the isolate was later identified as *N. asteroides.*

Bovine mammary gland infection with *Nocardia asteroides* was first reported from Australia in 1954 by Munch-Petersen.[15] Bovine mastitis due to *Nocardia* species was reported by Barnum and Fuller in Canada in 1956.[16] The first actinomycete definitely identified as *N. asteroides* from a bovine mammary gland infection in the United States was isolated the following year in Texas.[17]

Pier and fellow workers[18] made repeated isolations of *Nocardia asteroides* from milk where the infection was a problem on a herd basis. In a series of subsequent reports, the manifestations of the experimentally produced disease and the immunologic reactions of infected animals were recorded.[19,20] The oral infectivity and thermal resistance of the organism in milk was evaluated in a separate study.[21] Caprine mastitis caused by *N. asteroides* has been studied by Dafalla and Gharib in Africa.[22]

Nocardiosis has been diagnosed in marsupials,[23] but the identity of the species isolated was not established. *Nocardia asteroides* has been identified in infections in hatchery-reared fingerling rainbow trout (*Salmo gairdneri*).[24] The possibility that the fish were infected by the presence of the organism as a contaminant in pelleted food was considered.

Nocardia asteroides infections occur throughout the world. Most of the isolations to date have been made in Europe and the United States. On the basis of limited reports, *N. brasiliensis* and *N. caviae* have a more restricted geographic distribution. However, all have been found in soil, and they may be more widely distributed in nature than is presently recognized.

Several other aerobic actinomycetes cause subcutaneous and mycetoma type infections in man, but to date have not been reported from lower animals. These are *Nocardia madurae*, *Nocardia pelletieri*, and *Streptomyces somaliensis*. Until recently, all these species were in the genus *Streptomyces*, but studies of cell wall constituents have established a new criterion for differentiation. Members of the genus *Nocardia* contain a preponderance of mesodiaminopimelic acid in their cell walls; the major constituent in the cell wall of streptomycetes is LL-diaminopimelic acid.[25]

CLINICAL SIGNS AND PATHOLOGY

On original clinical examination, an impressive number of the cases of systemic nocardiosis described in dogs were tentatively diagnosed as distemper. This observation supports the statement of Ramsey and associates[26] that *Nocardia asteroides* has a notable predilection for the lungs and the central nervous system.

Most systemic canine nocardiosis cases have a history of two weeks or longer duration of the illness. The common signs are dyspnea, coughing, anorexia, and nasal and ocular discharges. A significant number have diarrhea which may be the result of general debility and sustained anorexia. The rectal temperature may vary between 102° and 104° F. Depression is common. During examination, one dog developed a "chewing gum" convulsion followed by incoordination.[27] In some cases, subcutaneous abscesses with draining sinuses are present, and enlarged, palpable lymph nodes may be detected.

Cutaneous and subcutaneous canine infections are much more common than systemic invasions. Many are not reported, particularly those that recover following therapy. Neal and Heath[28] have described a localized infection with a draining sinus in the popliteal region of the thigh. The sinus originated in the popliteal lymph node. The diagnosis was confirmed by cultural identification of *Nocardia asteroides*. Unfortunately, many recorded cases are not culturally confirmed.

The tissue response to invasion by *Nocardia* spp. is characteristically suppurative

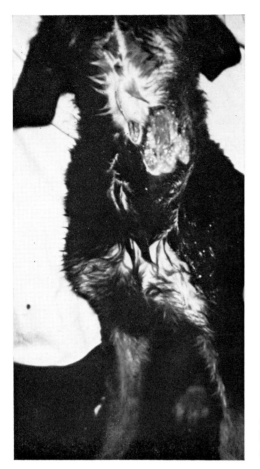

Fig. 12–1. Eroded subcutaneous abscess caused by *Nocardia aster-oides*. Multiple sinus tracts originated in cervical and prescapular lymph nodes.

Fig. 12–2. Nocardiosis. **A.** This photograph from a microabscess of the lung demonstrates the monotonous neutrophilic exudate which is the typical reaction in the majority of the lesions due to *Nocardia asteroides* that have been studied at the Armed Forces Institute of Pathology. No granules are seen. With the H & E. stain, no organisms are revealed. H & E. × 400. AFIP 657587 (60–1434). **B.** The branched filaments of *Nocardia asteroides* are well-shown in this photomicrograph of a slide stained by the Brown and Brenn Gram method. × 1350. (57–9743). **C.** The Gomori methenamine-silver stain demonstrates the filaments very well. × 1350. (57–9744). **D.** This photomicrograph of a slide was stained by Ziehl-Neelsen carbolfuchsin, decolorized with 1 percent aqueous sulfuric acid and photographed with use of a green filter. It shows the acid-fastness of the strain of *Nocardia asteroides* responsible for the lesions in this case. Acid-Fast Stain. × 1350. AFIP 680239 (57–13692). (Emmons, Binford and Utz, Medical Mycology, courtesy of Lea & Febiger)

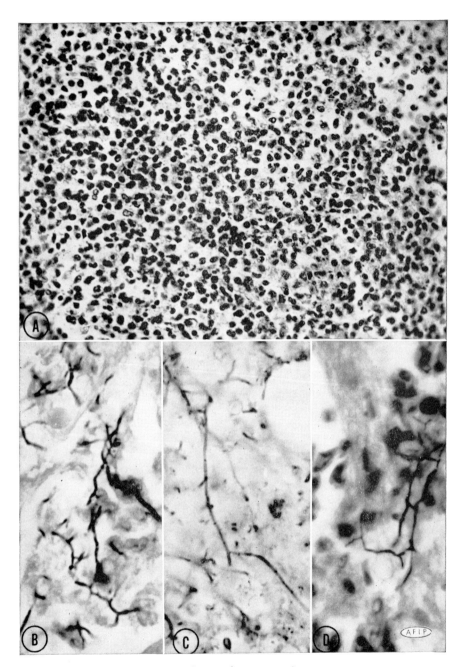

Fig. 12–2. Legend on opposite page.

and granulomatous. At necropsy, the lesions in the dog often are confined to the thoracic cavity. Serosanguineous fluid of varying amounts may be observed, and in the majority of cases a hemorrhagic pleuritis is present. The inflammatory and exudative proliferation may cover the pleura to a depth varying from one-fourth to two inches in thickness.[14] Abscesses or nodules, which may be discrete or confluent, occur in the pleura, lungs, myocardium and lymph nodes. In some generalized infections, similar lesions are seen in the subcutaneous tissue, spleen, liver, kidneys, mesenteric nodes and muscles. The pus in the abscesses is often fluid in consistency and is yellowish-grey in color.

Microscopic examination shows the lesions as tangled, indistinct colonies of organisms surrounded by necrotic cellular debris, purulent exudate and granulation tissue. Peripheral clubbing, as occurs in actinomycosis, usually is not seen. The organisms can be demonstrated in the tissues as gram-positive, branching filaments. They are not satisfactorily demonstrated in the usual hematoxylin and eosin preparations. The hyphae can usually be positively stained by the Brown and Breen or MacCallum-Goodpasture modifications of the Gram stain. The Gomori methenamine silver stain is satisfactory also.

The histologic picture of suppuration and granulation is markedly similar in different animal species and different anatomic sites. The similarity is consistent also between the pathogenic *Nocardia* spp. This is well-illustrated in the detailed descriptions of abscessation and necrosis surrounded by granulation reactions in feline nocardiosis caused by *N. brasiliensis*,[11] canine nocardiosis caused by *N. caviae*[12] and pulmonary nocardiosis caused by *N. asteroides* in the Rhesus monkey (*Macaca mulatta*).[29]

Bovine nocardiosis occurs chiefly as an infection of mammary tissue. Most infections are caused by *Nocardia asteroides*. In a few cases, *N. caviae* has been identified.[30] An isolate from mastitic milk reported as *N. brasiliensis* was identified later as *N. asteroides*.[11] In most cases, infection is confined to the mammary glands; usually only one quarter is involved. Occasionally the infection may metastasize to the supramammary and inguinal lymph nodes. Dissemination of the organism with the production of lesions in the lungs and other body organs may occur in natural acute infections or following experimental intramammary inoculation.[31]

Acute nocardial mastitis is often complicated with other mammary pathogens, particularly *Staphylococcus aureus*, *Corynebacterium pyogenes* or *Pseudomonas aeruginosa*. The disease is usually encountered in a single individual in a herd, but sometimes is seen as a serious herd problem. The degree of the infection varies from mild to severe but often shows uniformity within a herd.[31]

The clinical syndrome in acute nocardial mastitis is remarkably similar to the disease caused by mammary infection with toxin producing bacteria. The onset is sudden and usually closely follows parturition. The rectal temperature varies from 104° to 107° F., and dehydration is rapid. Severe depression, anorexia and complete cessation of milk flow are characteristic signs. Mammary secretions from infected glands may be viscid or watery and contain white or yellow flakes or granules. Blood clots may be evident also.

The affected mammary glands are enlarged and inflamed. Fibrosis and induration are apparent in 24 to 48 hours after onset. Subcutaneous nodules are often palpable. These may rupture to form draining sinus tracts. Occasionally an affected quarter will rupture. Deaths are not uncommon.

Chronic mastitis may follow mild and transitory clinical signs or occur in the animal that survives acute infection. In the former instance, the gland may become inflamed periodically and secrete abnormal milk. Fibrosis of the gland is slowly progressive as is loss of function.

At necropsy, the mammary gland is grossly enlarged and firm. Serosanguineous and purulent exudates appear on the incised surface. Areas of necrosis are usually apparent and palpable abscesses may be present in the secretory tissue. The gland cistern and teat sinus linings are thickened and covered with proliferative tissue.

LABORATORY DIAGNOSIS

Because of the environment in which many animals are kept, contamination of exudates and specimens submitted to a veterinary diagnostic laboratory is a common problem. The nocardiae are known to be present in soil, and the writer has made isolations in the laboratory which were considered to be contaminants.

Direct Microscopic Examination

Collect milk, pus, and spinal or other body fluids aseptically. These may be centrifuged for direct examination. Examine for granules in the pus from localized or mycetoma type infections. They are whitish in color and vary from 15 to 200 μ in size. They are not found in mastitic milk or in systemic nocardiosis.

Smears of the pus and centrifuged sediments should be stained with both the Gram and cold Kinyoun acid-fast methods using one percent aqueous sulfuric acid for decolorization in the latter method. Mycelial filaments stained by Gram's method stain irregularly and appear as long or branched hyphae less than one μ in diameter. The gram-positive filaments may appear "beaded" due to irregular staining or may appear as bacillary or coccobacillary elements. Likewise, in acid-fast stained smears, only parts of the hyphae may stain and bacillary or cocco-bacillary elements may be seen.

Culture

Clinical materials should be obtained aseptically and be submitted to the laboratory in sterile containers. Sabouraud's dextrose agar is a satisfactory isolation medium. The nocardiae may be sensitive to antibacterial antibiotics and these should not be added to the media. In routine culturing of mastitic milk, pure cultures are sometimes obtained on blood agar. However, because mixed infections and contaminants can be troublesome, Sabouraud's agar should be used simultaneously. These fungi grow more slowly than bacteria, and plates should be held for at least 96 hours before discarding as negative.

Agar plates or slants should be incubated at both room temperature and 37° C. Some strains of nocardiae grow poorly at room temperature. Many strains of *Nocardia asteroides* will withstand incubation at 50° C. Incubation at temperatures above 37° C. may prevent bacterial contaminants from growing.

Generally, the nocardial pathogens are slow growing. On blood agar, growth may not be apparent for 48 to 72 hours. They may develop even more slowly on Sabouraud's agar, particularly at room temperature. They develop to a diameter of five to ten mm. in 14–21 days. Colonial morphology varies greatly from flat and

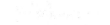

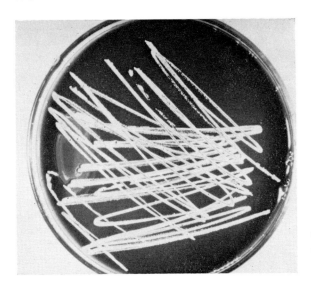

Fig. 12–3. White, chalky, adherent colonies of N. *asteroides* on blood agar after 96 hours incubation at 37° C.

glabrous to raised and wrinkled. The texture varies from smooth and soft or waxy and friable to chalky and hard. Color may vary from white or beige to yellow or yellowish-orange and occasionally red. Most isolates are glabrous at first, later developing a fine, powdery aerial mycelium. This feature is quite variable also; some develop only small amounts, others become completely covered and appear powdery or velvety.

Moist, smooth isolates of nocardiae may resemble bacterial colonies and may be difficult to distinguish from filamentous bacteria, particularly saprophytic mycobacteria. They may be differentiated by the strong acid-fastness of mycobacteria and their lack of true branching. The slide culture technique is excellent for demonstrating the filaments and true branching of *Nocardia* spp. Dry or "chalky" strains of nocardiae may resemble *Streptomyces* spp. morphologically. The filaments of both may terminally fragment into bacillary or coccoid spores. *Streptomyces* spp. are not acid-fast and may be differentiated by biochemical tests also.

Culture isolates should be stained by Gram's method and the modified cold Kinyoun acid-fast technique using one percent aqueous sulfuric acid for decolorization. Gram staining reveals Gram positive bacillary and coccoid forms. Some mycelial elements stain unevenly and appear "beaded." Since the hyphae are quite fragile, long filaments and branching usually are not seen. The distinguishing forms are seen when preparations are made from liquid or from slide cultures.

Nocardia asteroides, *N. brasiliensis* and *N. caviae* are partially acid-fast. This characteristic is somewhat variable. On initial isolation, young cultures usually are strongly acid-fast, but as the culture ages or is repeatedly transferred this quality diminishes. Growth of the organism in milk may partially or completely restore acid-fastness.

Gordon and her associates have made a series of studies of stable differential characteristics of pathogenic species of the genera *Streptomyces* and *Nocardia*.[30,32] In a recent report, she included the results of extensive studies of physiologic and biochemical properties of six pathogenic species.[33] Ajello and Basom[34] have tabulated some diagnostic properties of these species.

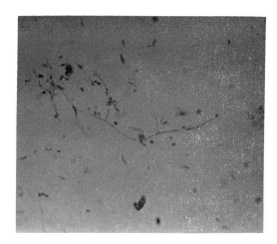

Fig. 12–4. Culture growth of *Nocardia asteroides*, Gram stain.

TABLE 12–1. Diagnostic Features of Actinomycotic Granules

Species	Color	Size	Tinctorial Reactions
N. asteroides*	Whitish	15–200 μ	Mycelium in granules of these three species acid - fast; hematoxylin - positive particles found within granules
N. brasiliensis*	Whitish	15–200μ	
N. caviae*	Whitish	15–200 μ	
N. madurae	Whitish	2–10 MM	Non-acid-fast; periphery hematoxylin positive
N. pelletieri	Pink to Red	150–500 μ	Non-acid-fast; entire grain hematoxylin positive
S. somaliensis	Whitish	0.5–2 MM	Non-acid-fast; entire grain hematoxylin negative

* Granules of these three species indistinguishable from each other.
Ajello, L., and Basom, W. C.: Dermatol. Internat., 7 (1968): 17–22. Courtesy J. B. Lippincott Company.

TABLE 12–2. Diagnostic Properties of the Actinomycotic Mycetoma Agents

Species	Acid fastness	Casein digestion	Xanthine digestion	Hypoxanthine digestion	Acid production with arabinose	Acid production with xylose
N. asteroides	+	−	−	−	−	−
N. brasiliensis	+	+	−	+	−	−
N. caviae	+	−	+	+	−	−
N. madurae	−	+	−	+	+	+
N. pelletieri	−	+	−	+	−	−
S. somaliensis	−	+	−	−	−	−

Ajello, L. and Basom, W. C.: Dermatol. Internat., 7 (1968): 17–22. Courtesy J. B. Lippincott Company.

Pathogenicity Tests

Animal inoculations are neither necessary nor practical for the diagnosis of nocardiosis. Guinea pigs will succumb following intraperitoneal injection of many strains of the systemic nocardiae, particularly if the inoculum is supplemented with gastric mucin. This is a fairly reliable method for obtaining tissues and exudates for classroom study.

Immunology

Skin test antigens and serologic tests are not available for the diagnosis of nocardiosis at present. Pier and associates have prepared an antigen from several strains of *N. asteroides.* They considered it to be a specific indicator of present or previous nocardiosis of cattle.[35]

DIFFERENTIAL DIAGNOSIS

Canine nocardiosis needs differentiation from distemper, encephalitis, rabies and pulmonary mycoses. Bovine nocardial mastitis has no distinct characteristics which differentiate it from acute or chronic mastitis caused by a variety of bacterial pathogens.

EPIDEMIOLOGY

Pathogenic nocardiae have been isolated from soil in many parts of the world. *Nocardia asteroides* has a wide geographic distribution, and it has been isolated from soil by many workers.[18,36,37] A preponderance of infections are caused by this species. *N. brasiliensis* and *N. caviae* apparently are less widely distributed. They are rarely identified as animal pathogens, and soil isolations are very rare.[33] *Nocardia asteroides* grows through a wide temperature range. This organism will withstand a temperature of 50° C. for several hours which enables it to survive and grow in composting vegetation.

Localized and mycetoma type infections follow injury to the skin and mucous membranes. Pulmonary infections result from inhalation of the organism. Systemic and cerebral infections follow hematogenous dissemination, usually from a primary pulmonary focus.

In mastitis, the organism gains entrance to the gland via the teat canal. *Nocardia asteroides* has been found in soil of dairy cattle holding pens.[18] The infection may be spread with contaminated infusion canulae. The presence of this fungus in milk has been a cause of concern because of potential danger to consumers. A study by Pier and Enright[21] of the thermal resistance of *N. asteroides* in milk has shown that it will not survive pasteurization.

Nocardial infections of man and animals have a common source in the soil. Nocardiosis is not transmitted from individual to individual or from animals to man.

TREATMENT

The nocardiae are gram-positive, and *in vitro* sensitivity tests often reveal them to be sensitive generally to the antibiotics effective against gram-positive bacteria. However, they often have questionable efficacy when evaluated by animal protection tests. Also, because antibiotics may enhance mycotic infections, many clinicians believe they are contraindicated in nocardiosis.

Sulfonamides are the drugs of choice in canine infections.[38,39] Sulfadiazine usually is well-tolerated, particularly if given in weekly interrupted courses. The dosage should be adequate to maintain blood levels no lower than 10 mg./100 ml. of blood. One-half to one gram orally four times daily is usually adequate. Supplemental iodide therapy may be helpful and may be given concurrently or during the periods of interruption of sulfonamide medication.

Actinomycotic (nocardial) mycetoma in man has been successfully treated with triple sulfa (sulfadiazine, sulfamerazine, sulfamethazine).[40] Two grams were given orally in four divided doses. Blood levels were maintained between 8 to 12 mg./100 ml.

Recently, Hoeprich and colleagues[41] have reported using cycloserine and sulfonamides to cure a nocardial brain abscess in a human patient. Treatment was continued over a period of several months.

Treatment of choice for bovine nocardial mastitis is sulfonamides also, or sulfonamides supplemented with nitrofurazone. Pier and associates[42] have reported on the use of a combination of nitrofurazone and novobiocin. The previously mentioned objection to use of antibiotics in these infections should be considered.

Sanitation and good milking practices are more important than chemotherapy in control of nocardiosis in a herd. A long rest period between lactations may be more helpful than therapy. Chlorine, 100 parts per million (p.p.m.) for five minutes or 100 p.p.m. benzalkonium chloride for ten minutes is fungicidal for nocardiae.

The antifungal antibiotics—nystatin, amphotericin B and griseofulvin—have no therapeutic value in the treatment of nocardiosis.[43]

REFERENCES

1. Nocard, E.: Note sur la Maladie des Boeufs de la Guadaloupe Connue sous le Nom de farcin. Ann. Inst. Pasteur, *2* (1888): 293–302.
2. Gordon, R. E. and Mihm, J. M.: The Type Species of the Genus *Nocardia*. J. Gen. Microbiol., *27* (1962): 1–10.
3. Eppinger, H.: Ueber eine neue Pathogene Cladothrix und eine durch sie hervorgernfene Pseudotuberculosis. Wien. klin. Wschr., *3* (1890): 221.
4. Breed, R. S., Murray, E. G. D. and Smith, N. R.: *Bergey's Manual of Determinative Bacteriology*. 7th edition, Baltimore, Williams & Wilkins Co., 1957.
5. Gordon, R. E. and Mihm, J. M.: A Comparative Study of Some Strains Received as *Nocardia*. J. Bact., *73* (1957): 15–27.
6. Hathaway, B. M. and Mason, K. N.: Nocardiosis—Study of Fourteen Cases. Amer. J. Med., *32* (1962): 903–909.
7. Balozet, L. and Pernot, P.: Meningite du Chien Causee par un Actinomyces. Bull. Acad. Vet. France, *9* (1936): 168–177.
8. Ginsberg, A. and Little, A. C. W.: Actinomycosis in Dogs. J. Path. Bac., *60* (1948): 563–572.
9. Bohl, E. H., Jones, D. O., Farrell, R. L., Chamberlain, D. M., Cole, C. R. and Ferguson, L. C.: Nocardiosis in the Dog: A Case Report. J. Amer. Vet. Med. Ass., *122* (1953): 81–85.
10. Maddy, K. T., Stroud, M. E. and Ajello, L.: Nocardiosis in the Dog: A Case Report. Vet. Med., *9* (1955): 414–416.
11. Ajello, L., Walker, W. W., Dungworth, D. L. and Brumfield, G. L.: Isolation of *Nocardia brasiliensis* from a Cat. J. Amer. Vet. Med. Ass., *138* (1961): 370–376.
12. Kinch, D. A.: A Rapidly Fatal Infection Caused by *Nocardia caviae* in a Dog. J. Path. Bac., *95* (1968): 540–546.
13. Mostafa, I. E., Cerny, L. and Cerna, J.: Canine Nocardiosis due to *Nocardia caviae*. Abs. No. 2248. Rev. Med. Vet. Mycol. *6* (1969): 462.
14. Langham, R. F., Schirmer, R. G. and Newman, J. P.: Nocardiosis in the Dog and Cat. M.S.U. Vet., *19* (1959): 102–108.

15. Munch-Petersen, E.: *Actinomyces (Nocardia) sp.* from a Bovine Udder Infection. Aust. Vet. J., *30* (1954): 297–300.

16. Barnum, D. A. and Fuller, D. S.: A Report on the Isolation of Two Species of Nocardia from Bovine Mastitis. Ann. Meet. Northeast Mastitis Coun., St. Hyacinthe, Quebec, Canada, Oct., 1956.

17. Jungerman, P : Fungus Mastitis: A Case Report. Vet. Med., *53* (1958): 53–54.

18. Pier, A. C., Gray, D. M. and Fossatti, M. J.: *Nocardia asteroides*—A Newly Recognized Pathogen of the Mastitis Complex. Amer. J. Vet. Res., *19* (1958): 319–331.

19. Pier, A. C., Willers, E. H. and Mejia, M. J.: *Nocardia asteroides* as a Mammary Pathogen of Cattle. II. The Sources of Nocardial Infection and Experimental Reproduction of the Disease. Amer. J. Vet. Res., *22* (1961): 698–703.

20. Pier, A. C., and Enright, J. B.: *Nocardia asteroides* as a Mammary Pathogen of Cattle. III. Immunologic Reactions of Infected Animals. Amer. J. Vet. Res., *23* (1962): 284–292.

21. Pier, A. C. and Enright, J. B.: Oral Infectivity and Thermal Resistance of *Nocardia asteroides* in Milk. Public Health Rep., *76* (1961): 889–895.

22. Dafalla, E. N. and Gharib, H. M.: A Study of Mastitis in a Goat Caused by *Nocardia asteroides*. Brit. Vet. J., *114* (1958): 143–145.

23. Tucker, R. and Millar, R.: Outbreak of Nocardiosis in Marsupials in the Brisbane Botanical Gardens. J. Comp. Path. Ther., *63* (1953): 143–146.

24. Snieszko, S. F., Bullock, G. L., Dunbar, C. E. and Pettijohn, L. L.: Nocardial Infection in Hatchery-Reared Fingerling Rainbow Trout (*Salmo gairdneri*), J. Bact., *88* (1964): 1809–1810.

25. Becker, B., Lechevalier, M. P., Gordon, R. and Lechevalier, H. A.: Rapid Differentiation Between *Nocardia* and *Streptomyces* by Paper Chromatography of Whole-Cell Hydrolysates. Appl. Microbiol., *12* (1964): 421–423.

26. Ramsey, F. K., Brandner, C. R. and Baker, D. L.: Nocardiosis in a Dog. Iowa St. Col. Vet., *14* (1957): 173–176.

27. Rhoades, H. E., Reynolds, H. A., Rahm, D. P. and Small, E.: Nocardiosis in a Dog with Multiple Lesions of the Central Nervous System. J. Amer. Med. Vet. Ass., *142* (1963): 278–281.

28. Neal, J. E. and Heath, M. K.: Nocardiosis in Dogs. Auburn Vet., *11* (1955): 112–114.

29. Jonas, A. M. and Wyand, D. S.: Pulmonary Nocardiosis in the Rhesus Monkey. Path. Vet., *3* (1966): 588–600.

30. Gordon, R. E. and Mihm, J. M.: Identification of *Nocardia caviae* (Erickson) *nov. comb.* Ann. N.Y. Acad. Sci., *98* (1962): 628–636.

31. Pier, A. C., Mejia, M. J. and Willers, E. H.: *Nocardia asteroides* as a Mammary Pathogen of Cattle. I. The Disease in Cattle and the Comparative Virulence of 5 Isolates. Amer. J. Vet. Res., *22* (1961): 502–517.

32. Gordon, R. E. and Smith, M. M.: Proposed Group of Characters for the Separation of Streptomyces and Nocardia. J. Bact., *69* (1955): 147–150.

33. Gordon, R. E.: Some Criteria for the Recognition of *Nocardia madurae* (Vincent) Blanchard. J. Gen. Microbiol., *45* (1966): 355–364.

34. Ajello, L. and Basom, W. C.: A Mexican Case of Mycetoma Caused by *Streptomyces somaliensis*. Dermatol. Internal., *7* (1968): 17–22.

35. Pier, A. C., Thurston, J. R. and Larsen, A. B.: A Diagnostic Antigen for Nocardiosis: Comparative Tests in Cattle with Nocardiosis and Mycobacteriosis. Amer. J. Vet. Res., *29* (1968): 397–403.

36. Gordon, R. E. and Hagen, W. A.: A Study of Some Acid-Fast Actinomycetes from Soil with Special Reference to Pathogenicity for Animals. J. Infect. Dis., *59* (1936): 200–206.

37. Emmons, C. W.: The Significance of Saprophytism in the Epidemiology of the Mycoses. Trans. N. Y. Acad. Sci., *17* (1954): 157–166.

38. Swerczek, T. W., Trautwein, G. and Nielsen, S. W.: Canine Nocardiosis. Zbl. Vet. Med., *15* (B, 1968): 971–978.

39. Wolff, E. F.: Canine Nocardiosis—A Case Report and Literature Review. Southern Vet., *6* (1969): 4–8.

40. Bergeron, J. R., Mullins, J. F. and Ajello, L.:   Mycetoma Caused by *Nocardia pelletieri* in the United States. Arch. Derm., *99* (1969): 564–566.
41. Hoeprich, P. D., Brandt, D. and Parker, R. H.:   Nocardial Brain Abscess Cured with Cycloserine and Sulfonamides.   Amer. J. Med. Sci., *225* (1968): 208–215.
42. Pier, A. C., Gray, D. M and Fossatti, M. J.:   *Nocardia asteroides*—A Newly Recognized Pathogen of the Mastitis Complex.   Amer. J. Vet. Res., *19* (1958): 319–331.
43. Hilick-Smith, G., Blank, H. and Imrich, S.:   *Fungus Diseases and Their Treatment.* Boston, Little, Brown & Co., 1964.

CHAPTER 13 | Dermatophilosis

Dermatophilosis, caused by the aerobic and facultatively anaerobic actinomycete *Dermatophilus congolensis*, is an ulcerative, cutaneous disease of man and several species of lower animals. It is commonly called "cutaneous streptothricosis" and "mycotic dermatitis." The disease is usually chronic and it may cause important economic losses.

HISTORY, GEOGRAPHIC DISTRIBUTION AND PREVALENCE

Van Saceghem,[1] in 1915, first described dermatophilosis as a specific disease of cattle in the former Belgian Congo, and he named the causative organism *Dermatophilus congolensis*. Subsequently he described the fungus in culture and stated that sheep, goats and horses can be infected with *D. congolensis* but less severely than cattle.[2]

In the decade following Van Saceghem's original report, the disease was discovered and was found to be enzootic in several countries in Africa. Sporadic cases were discovered in New Zealand, Australia and India.[3] Bridges and Romane[4] first reported the disease in the United States in 1961 in Texas cattle. In the same year, Dean[5] disclosed infections in four people who had handled an infected deer in New York, and Bentinck-Smith and associates[6] described the disease in 15 horses from New York and Vermont. More recently, bovine and equine cases have been discovered in Iowa, Kansas and Georgia.[7,8,9]

A confusing synonymy has evolved for both the disease syndrome and its causal agent. Dermatophilosis is known by many different names in cattle, horses, sheep and goats. Some are descriptive of clinical signs or local lesions in their respective hosts. In a comprehensive review, Szabuniewicz has arranged them both chronologically and within animal species.[3] Currently, dermatophilosis is commonly called "cutaneous streptothricosis" when it affects cattle, horses, goats, deer and man. In sheep, when wool-covered areas of the body are invaded, the terms "lumpy wool," "rain rot," or "mycotic dermatitis" are applied. Inflammatory and exudative lesions of the distal extremities and coronet in sheep are known as "proliferative dermatitis" or "strawberry foot rot" and to date have been reported from Scotland only. For the sake of clarity, all infections caused by *Dermatophilus congolensis* should be called dermatophilosis.

Early workers incorrectly placed the causative organism in several different genera (*Streptothrix*, *Actinomyces*, *Nocardia* and *Polysepta*).[10] Until recently, in addition to *Dermatophilus congolensis*, two other species, *Dermatophilus dermatonomous* and *D. pedis*, were recognized as causing ovine "mycotic dermatitis" and "strawberry foot rot," respectively. Gordon has studied all three "species" comprehensively and concluded that they are the same. Thus, *D. congolensis* is the valid name on the basis of priority with *D. dermatonomous* and *D. pedis* in synonymy.[11]

Well-authenticated cases have been recorded in cattle, horses, sheep, goats, deer and man. The disease has been found in zebra, antelope and eland in Africa. Reports of dermatophilosis in hogs,[12] cats[13] and the turkey[14] are questionable. Either cultural confirmation is lacking or histopathologic data suggest the probability of infection by a different etiologic agent.

Like many other mycotic diseases, dermatophilosis was first thought to be tropical and exotic. It is known now to have worldwide distribution. Although not reported in North America until recent years, it is rapidly becoming evident that it is widespread there also. Recently animal cases were found in Florida[15] and in Ontario,[16] Canada. The disease is probably more prevalent than is recognized even now. Veterinarians and laboratorians should become familiar with the disease and its etiologic agent.

CLINICAL SIGNS AND PATHOLOGY

The early cutaneous lesions of bovine dermatophilosis may be barely visible but easily detected by running the fingers over affected areas. Close examination may show small vesicles, and papules, or edema and pus formation under "gummy" hair plaques. Soon an exudative dermatitis appears which is characterized by multiple raised areas in which the hair is erect and matted with exudates into tufts which resemble the tip of a fine paint brush.[3]

As the disease progresses, the exudates coalesce to form yellowish brown scabs which, in turn, change to hard crusts firmly adherent to the skin. The crusts enlarge, become elevated and hardened, and resemble hyperkeratosis. In some

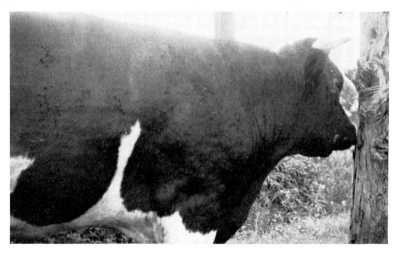

Fig. 13-1. Early lesions of bovine dermatophilosis. Note similarity to lesions of exanthema nodularis bovis shown in Fig. 13-5. (Courtesy of Dr. M. Szabuniewicz)

13

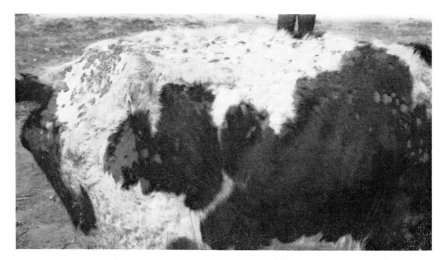

Fig. 13–2. Lesions of cow caused by *Dermatophilus congolensis*. (Courtesy of
Dr. M. Szabuniewicz)

instances, hair may be retained in the crust, or large, fairly circumscribed scabs may
completely obscure the hair.   Individual scabs may attain a diameter of several
inches.   When healing occurs, the scabs slough off, and new hair may appear or
alopecic signs may persist.

Equine dermatophilosis most commonly affects areas of the back, sides or rump.
Less often the neck, head or legs are affected.   Kaplan and Johnston[9] observed
lesions on all parts of the body except the thorax and abdomen.   One horse they
described had large coalesced lesions covering the length of the back and extending
down over the side and shoulder.   They described early equine lesions as irregular
patches of matted hair or as raised crusted areas, with hairs protruding through the
crusts.   In severely affected animals, the crusts were separated from the underlying
skin.   On removal of the crusts, a moist pink area or soft smooth skin was observed.

Ovine dermatophilosis may be so mild that the herdsman is not aware of the
infection other than a loss of wool.   Occasionally only scabby lesions will be observed on the ears and nose, particularly in lambs.   Hart[17] has described varying
degrees of severity for infection in sheep and graded them by numerical scores.
Score one infections showed erythema, papule formation or, more commonly,
localized exudation or isolated flecks of white, yellow or brown solid grease or
crust.   The latter sometimes bound small groups of wool fibers together.   Score
two was assigned when there was sufficient exudate or crust to bind larger and more
numerous bundles of wool fibers together.   More severe erythema and papule
formation were included in this score.   Score three exudates were either moist or
dry and varied in color.   These covered large areas and were palpable.   Wool was
damaged.   Score four infections had larger and thicker crusts than score three.
Score five crusts were extremely hard, dense or hornlike.   The number and severity
of Hart's cases were related to seasonal weather changes, both increasing in wet
weather.

Austwick and Davies[18] have described occasional intense, transient pruritus which
caused the animals to rub under fences and sometimes to gnaw at their flanks pro-

ducing raw, profusely bleeding areas. Intense pruritus is not a usual feature of bovine and equine infections.

Ovine "strawberry foot rot" appears to be widespread in Scotland. Its name is derived from the appearance of the lesions. If the scabs are removed, a number of bleeding points present themselves on a fleshy mass and the exposed lesion closely resembles a fresh strawberry. The condition is an ulcerative dermatitis affecting the skin of the legs from the coronet to above the knee or hock. Interestingly, Harris[19] in 1948 stated that the infection is transmissible to man, and this may be the first reference to human infection with *Dermatophilus congolensis*.

Histopathologic examination of skin sections shows the infection to be quite superficial. Mycelium of the fungus may be found in the keratinized epithelial cells and hair follicles, but not within the hair. Both branching and fragmented hyphae are often abundant in the surface exudates which are composed of keratinized epithelial cells, leucocytes and serum. Microabscesses are a consistent finding in the epidermis. The follicles may be plugged with mycelium, keratin and necrotic debris. The epithelial layer may be separated by accumulations of neutrophils and serous exudates. Changes in the dermis are characterized by mixed inflammatory cell infiltration.

LABORATORY DIAGNOSIS

The laboratory should request material from acute, active lesions if available. Tufts of hair with attached epidermal crusts, smears from exudates or pus, and smears from scrapings of active lesions should be submitted. The organisms are sparse and are often difficult to find in stained smears of chronic and healing lesions. Also, the chances of obtaining successful cultures are lessened with material from chronic lesions.

Direct Microscopic Examination

Make additional thick smears from the moist undersurface of epithelial crusts and scabs. Most workers obtain best results with Giemsa stain. However, methylene blue or Wright's stain may be useful. Pier and co-workers[7] recommend Giemsa stain for 30 minutes to an hour followed by acid alcohol decolorization. This procedure removes excess stain from the smear and aids the search for the organism which has a strong stain affinity.

Examine under oil immersion for branching hyphae which may be intact or fragmented. Intact hyphae initially are approximately one μ in diameter. Fragmentation occurs first transversely to form coccoid or disclike "spores." Longitudinal division then occurs and packets are formed of two to eight rows of parallel coccoid cells. After longitudinal division, the filaments may have a diameter of 3.5 μ. These parallel rows of coccoid bodies in one filament are substantiative evidence of dermatophilosis.

Culture

Clinical material may be streaked directly onto suitable solid media or first may be pulverized in a mortar, diluted with saline, and then inoculated. The organism requires a rich culture medium such as blood agar or BHI agar. It will not grow on Sabouraud dextrose agar or on agar containing most antibiotics.

Most writers have mentioned difficulty in obtaining isolations because of over-

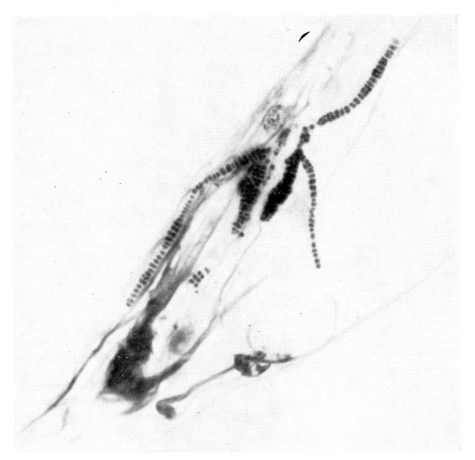

Fig. 13–3. Giemsa stain of *Dermatophilus congolensis* in pus and exudate from cow in former Belgian Congo. (Courtesy of Dr. M. Szabuniewicz)

growth of the colonies by contaminants. This problem may be alleviated by the use of azide blood agar for primary isolation. A disadvatnage with this medium is that colonies of *Dermatophilus congolensis* do not appear until postinoculation day four.[20]

Haalstra[21] has described a relatively dependable technique for isolation of *Dermatophilus congolensis* from clinical materials. His method is based on Roberts' study of the release of zoospores after moistening and on chemotaxis of the motile zoospores to carbon dioxide.[22] Small pieces of scabs or crusts are placed in small bottles or tubes. One ml. distilled water is added and the specimens are held for three and one-half hours at room temperature. The specimens are then placed in a candle jar for 15 minutes. Samples of the surface water are taken with a bacteriologic loop and inoculated onto blood agar or BHI agar plates. The plates are incubated in a candle jar at 37° C. for 24 to 48 hours. Overgrowth with contaminants usually is not a problem. After 24–36 hours' incubation, characteristic colonies have a "lacelike" fimbriated appearance peripherally and are slightly *beta*-hemolytic on blood agar. Typical colonies are greyish white in color, raised, rough and

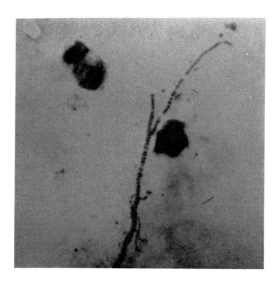

Fig. 13–4. Gram stain of *Derma-tophilus congolensis* cultured from scab material of horse.

0.5–1.0 mm. in diameter. Older colonies enlarge to 4 or more mm. in diameter, become yellow to orange in color, usually are depressed in the agar and are quite adherent. Variant strains in both color and texture have been described by Gordon.[11]

Smears of the cultures may be Gram-stained, but Giemsa stain usually portrays the elements more sharply. Depending upon the age of the cultures, microscopic examination reveals the various developmental stages of the organism identical to the forms found in infected tissue. In young colonies, narrow branching septate hyphae are formed. On continued growth, the hyphae divide first transversely, then longitudinally, and by 72–96 hours the hyphae may attain a diameter of 3–5 μ and contain packets up to eight coccoid cells in width. Under conditions suitable for continued growth, these packets eventually break up and release motile coccoid zoospores. The flagellated zoospores subsequently can germinate and produce germ tubes that will develop into branched, septate hyphae.

Dermatophilus congolensis is gram-positive and non-acid-fast. This organism produces acid in dextrose and fructose within 48 hours. Slight to distinct acid is produced in maltose in one or two weeks. Acid is not produced from dulcitol, lactose, mannitol, salicin, sorbitol or xylose. Gas is not produced in the carbo-hydrates. Urea is hydrolyzed in 24 hours, and catalase is produced within five days. Nitrate is not reduced, nor is indol formed. The organism is methyl red and Voges-Proskauer negative. Strain variations in proteolytic properties have recently been recorded by Gordon.[11]

Pathogenicity Tests

In addition to rabbits, *Dermatophilus congolensis* is pathogenic for guinea pigs and mice. However, pathogenicity tests are not necessary to identify the organism.

Immunology

It has not been established if recovery from dermatophilosis in cattle and horses confers protection against subsequent reinfection. Szabuniewicz (personal com-munication) has observed a large number of cases during several years in Africa without recalling a single reinfection. Many of the cases he diagnosed were in dairies under close observation. On the other hand, he saw untreated cattle which had been affected for longer than two years. This, considered with the fact that infection does not cause a marked inflammatory response in the host indicates that immunity, if any, is minimal.

Roberts[23] has studied the effect of circulating antibody in sheep, and he stated that acquired resistance is due to an enhancement by antibody of the destructive phase of phagocytosis. He also advanced the possibility of the severe inflammatory lesions of "strawberry foot rot" being an allergic reaction.

Gordon[11] has demonstrated common precipitinogens in all *Dermatophilus congolensis* strains tested, and he produced specific precipitin antibodies in sheep, goats and rabbits. Serum from the goat did not cross react with *Nocardia asteroides* or *Actinomyces bovis* antigens.

Pier and colleagues[24] have successfully used the fluorescent antibody technique to demonstrate *Dermatophilus congolensis* in clinical materials.

DIFFERENTIAL DIAGNOSIS

The clinical signs of bovine scabies and dermatophilosis, particularly in early stages, are quite similar. These two diseases may occur simultaneously.[25] Dermatophilosis may need differentiation from warts and from infection with *Trichophyton verrucosum*. Cases with extensive lesions may resemble photosensitization, urticaria, hyperkeratosis and cutaneous besnoitiosis. In Africa and South America, lumpy skin disease (exanthema nodularis bovis) should be considered also. In lambs, dermatophilosis may resemble "orf" (contagious pustular dermatitis).

EPIDEMIOLOGY

To date, the only isolations of *Dermatophilus congolensis* have been from lesions of affected animals and man. It is unknown if the organism can exist in nature.

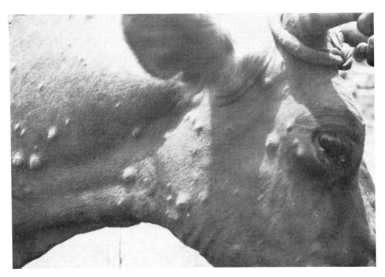

Fig. 13–5. Bovine lumpy skin disease (exanthema nodularis bovis). (Courtesy of Dr. M. Szabuniewicz)

Efforts to recover the fungus from soil in habitats of infected animals have failed,[9] and studies have shown that the organism cannot survive for long periods in soil, particularly when exposed to moisture.[26]

It is not known if the organism is transmitted from animal to animal by direct contact or if vectors spread the disease. Dermatophilosis has been experimentally transmitted from infected to normal rabbits in the laboratory by flies,[27] but it has not been proven if this method of transmission occurs in nature.

Many workers believe that *Dermatophilus congolensis* can exist as a commensal on the skin of normal animals and that it becomes pathogenic only after predisposing factors alter the normal skin. Minor injuries, insect bites and prolonged wetting by rain have all been incriminated. Maceration of the skin by prolonged wetting is generally accepted as the most important predisposing factor. Also, wetting facilitates the release of infective zoospores and may provide the means of enhanced motility.

Humans have become infected after handling animals with dermatophilosis. However, in view of the number of persons in close contact with affected animals and the rare occurrence of animal-to-man transmission, it appears that the organism has a low order of pathogenicity for man.

TREATMENT

No single treatment regimen is considered specific for dermatophilosis. Many clinicians believe it is most important to remove the scabs, thus facilitating contact of the medication with the organisms. Szabuniewicz recommends use of stiff brush and mild soap solution.[3] Various topical agents have been used successfully. These include tincture of methyl violet, two-percent tincture of iodine, raw linseed oil and seven-percent tincture of iodine in equal parts, iodoform ointment, copper sulfate (1:500 aqueous solution), mercuric chloride-salicylic acid ointment, and many other proprietary antiparasitic, bactericidal and fungicidal formulations.

Dermatophilus congolensis is sensitive in vitro to many antibacterial antibiotics and sulfonamides. A combination of penicillin and streptomycin has given good therapeutic results in both bovine[20] and equine[16] infections. Roberts[28] has reported cures in sheep with penicillin alone. In all species, it is important that large doses be given and therapy be continued for several days. The effect of therapy is difficult to evaluate because some cases recover spontaneously without treatment.[8,16] Various dips have been used, particularly in sheep, both therapeutically and to control vectors. Copper sulfate is inexpensive but may affect dyeing qualities of the wool.[29] One-half percent zinc sulfate has been recommended to prevent infections in shearing injuries.[28] Arsenicals and benzene hexachloride were reported to be helpful in controlling infections of cattle in Africa.[3]

Quarantine of affected animals is recommended to prevent possible spread of the disease by contact and vectors. Whenever possible, shelter should be provided to protect patients from rain and inclement weather.

REFERENCES

1. Van Saceghem, R.: Dermatose Contagieuse (Impetigo Contagieux). Bull. Soc. Path. Exot., *8* (1915): 354–359.
2. Van Saceghem, R.: Impetigo Contagieux et Impetigo Tropical. Bull. Agri. du Congo Belge, *25* (1935): 591–598.

3. Szabuniewicz, M.: Cutaneous Streptothricosis in Cattle. Southwest Vet., *18* (1964): 41–48.

4. Bridges, C. H. and Romane, W. M.: Cutaneous Streptothricosis in Cattle. J. Amer. Vet. Med. Ass., *138* (1961): 153–157.

5. Dean, D. J., Gordon, M. A., Severinghaus, C. W., Kroll, E. T. and Reilly, J. R.: Streptothricosis: A New Zoonotic Disease. New York J. Med., *61* (1961): 1283–1287.

6. Bentinck-Smith, J., Fox, F. H. and Baker, D. W.: Equine Dermatitis (Cutaneous Streptothricosis) Infection with Dermatophilus in the United States. Cornell Vet., *51* (1961): 334–339.

7. Pier, A. C., Neal, E. C. and Cysewski, S. J.: Cutaneous Streptothricosis in Iowa Cattle. J. Amer. Vet. Med. Ass., *142* (1963): 995–1000.

8. Kelley, D. C. and Knappenberger, T. E.: Cutaneous Streptothricosis (Equine Dermatophilosis) in Kansas Horses. Vet. Med., *63* (1968): 1055–1056.

9. Kaplan, W. and Johnston, W. J.: Equine Dermatophilosis (Cutaneous Streptothricosis) in Georgia. J. Amer. Vet. Med. Ass., *149* (1966): 1162–1171.

10. Ainsworth, G. C. and Austwick, P. K. C.: *Fungal Diseases of Animals.* Farnham Royal, Bucks, England, Commonwealth Agricultural Bureau, 1959.

11. Gordon, M. A.: The Genus Dermatophilus. J. Bact., *88* (1964): 509–522.

12. Vandemaele, F. P.: Enquette sur la Streptothricose Cutanee en Afrique. Bull. Epizoot. Dis. Afr., *3* (1961): 251–258.

13. O'Hara, P. J. and Cordes, D. O.: Granulomata Caused by Dermatophilus in Two Cats. New Zealand Vet. J., *11* (1963): 151–154.

14. Soliman, K. N. and Rellison, D. H. L.: Mycotic Infection of the Skin of the Turkey. Vet. Rec., *63* (1951): 20–24.

15. Tucker, W. E.: A Case Report of Cutaneous Streptothricosis in a Florida Bull. The Practicing Vet. (Pitman-Moore Division of Dow Chemical Company), (1966): 46.

16. Searcy, G. P. and Hulland, T. J.: Dermatophilus Dermatitis (Streptothricosis) in Ontario. I., Canad. Vet. J., *9* (1968): 7–15.

17. Hart, C. B.: Mycotic Dermatitis in Sheep. I. Clinical Observations in Great Britain. Vet. Rec., *81* (1967): 36–47.

18. Austwick, P. K. C. and Davies, E. T.: Mycotic Dermatitis in Great Britain. 1954–1958. Vet. Rec., *70* (1958): 1081–1088.

19. Harris, S. T.: Proliferative Dermatitis of the Legs ("Strawberry Foot Rot") in Sheep. J. Comp. Path. Ther., *58* (1948): 314–328.

20. Shotts, E. B., Jr., Tyler, D. E. and Christy, J. E.: Cutaneous Streptothricosis in a Bull. J. Amer. Vet. Med. Ass., *154* (1969): 1450–1454.

21. Haalstra, R. T.: Isolation of *Dermatophilus congolensis* from Skin Lesions in the Diagnosis of Streptothricosis. Vet. Rec., 77 (1965): 824–825.

22. Roberts, D. S.: Chemotactic Behavior of the Infective Zoospores of *Dermatophilus dermatonomous.* Aust. J. Agri. Res., *14* (1963): 400–411.

23. Roberts, D. S.: Dermatophilus Infection. Vet. Bull., *37* (1967): 513–521.

24. Pier, A. C., Richard, J. L. and Farrell, E. F.: Fluorescent Antibody and Cultural Techniques in Cutaneous Streptothricosis. Amer. J. Vet. Res., *25* (1964): 1014–1020.

25. Macadam, I.: Observations on the Effects of Flies and Humidity on the Natural Lesions of Streptothricosis. Vet. Rec., *76* (1964): 194–197.

26. Roberts, D. S.: The Release and Survival of *Dermatophilus dermatonomus* Zoospores. Aust. J. Agri. Res., *14* (1963): 386–399.

27. Richard, J. L. and Pier, A. C.: Transmission of *Dermatophilus congolensis* by *Stomoxys calcitrans* and *Musca domestica.* Amer. J. Vet. Res., *27* (1966): 419–423.

28. Roberts, D. S.: An Approach to the Control of Mycotic Dermatitis. Wool Tech. and Sheep Breeding, *9* (1962): 101–103.

29. Story, L. F.: Bluestone Absorbed by Wool Affects Processing. New Zeal. J. Agri., *85* (1952): 501–503.

Index

(Page numbers in *italics* refer to illustrations; page numbers followed by n refer to footnotes, and those followed by t, refer to tables)